Equalising Opportunities, Minimising Oppression

D0278367

Anti-Racist Practice (ARP), Anti-Discriminatory Practice (ADP), and Anti-Oppressive Practice (AOP), form a trinity of concepts, nested into one another, which have evolved in welfare services over the last fifteen years. They tend to have developed as forms of practice panaceas and as a result have been subject to both unrealistic expectations and, at times, to political ridicule. This book

- clarifies the distinctions between three key concepts – ARP, ADP and AOP
- critically and constructively analyses the three approaches to practice
- reappraises their potential in the light of emerging equality issues in the health service.

With contributions from leading teachers and practitioners in the field, covering all forms of equal opportunities: gender; ethnicity; disability; sexuality and age-related discriminations, *Equalising Opportunities, Minimising Oppression* provides students and practitioners in health and social care with a clear overview of an area where there is much confusion and imperfect understanding.

Dylan Ronald Tomlinson is an Educational Consultant. **Winston Trew** is a consultant in urban regeneration and capacity building.

Equalising Opportunities, Minimising Oppression

A critical review of anti-discriminatory policies in health and social welfare

Edited by Dylan Ronald Tomlinson and Winston Trew

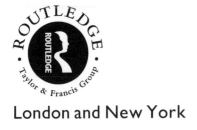

London and New York

First published 2002
by Routledge
11 New Fetter Lane, London EC4P 4EE

Simultaneously published in the USA and Canada
by Routledge
29 West 35th Street, New York, NY 10001

Routledge is an imprint of the Taylor & Francis Group

Typeset in Times and Gill by BC Typesetting, Bristol
Printed and bound in Malta by
Gutenberg Press Limited

British Library Cataloguing in Publication Data
A catalogue record for this book is available from the British Library

Library of Congress Cataloging in Publication Data
Equalising opportunities, minimising oppression: a critical review of
anti-disciminatory policies in health and social welfare/edited by
Dylan Ronald Tomlinson and Winston Trew.
    p. cm.
  Includes bibliographical references and index.
  1. Right to health care–Great Britain. 2. Public welfare–Great Britain.
3. Discrimination–Great Britain. I. Tomlinson, Dylan Ronald.
II. Trew, Winston.

R724.E684 2001
362.1'0941–dc21   2001052017

ISBN 0–415–25087–0 (pbk)
     0–415–25086–2 (hbk)

Contents

Contributors

Uduak Archibong, Ph.D. is Senior Lecturer in the School of Health Studies at the University of Bradford. Her main areas of work concern the development of methods to enhance levels of cross-cultural competence among health service practitioners, and she provides a 'Managing Diversity' training and consultation for both staff and students in academic and health care arenas.

Naaz Coker is Director of Race and Diversity/Education and Leadership at the King's Fund and Chair of the British Refugee Council. She has developed particular expertise in the area of health and diversity, drawing on many years' experience of clinical and general management roles in the NHS; she is editor of *Racism and Medicine* (2001, King's Fund).

Lena Dominelli, Ph.D. is Professor of Social Work at the University of Southampton and President of the International Association of Schools of Social Work. She is working on the development of a holistic approach to anti-oppressive practice and is the author of the forthcoming Palgrave text *Anti-Oppressive Practice: From Oppressive to Empowering Social Work*.

Geoffrey Mercer, Ph.D. is Senior Lecturer in Sociology at the University of Leeds Centre for Disability Studies. He has a particular interest in the growth of 'independent living' and the disabled people's movement, which are the subjects of his current research, and is the co-author, with Colin Barnes and Tom Shakespeare, of *Exploring Disability* (1999, Polity Press).

Rabbi Julia Neuberger is Chief Executive of the King's Fund and has extensive health service experience in the management of diversity issues. She has taken a particular interest in advocacy for the health and welfare of minority ethnic groups in the UK, and has recently established a range of projects at the King's Fund which reflect that concern.

Naina Patel, OBE is the Director and founder of PRIAE, the Policy Research Institute on Ageing and Ethnicity, established in 1998 as the first body of its kind in Europe. The author of many social work texts, most recently contributing to *Beyond Racial Divides – Ethnicities in Social Work Practice* (2001, Routledge), Naina has also produced films about race and equal opportunities.

Gurnam Singh is Senior Lecturer in Social Work at Coventry University where he is a founder member of the Centre for Social Justice. He is a contributor to the Routledge (1998) book *Social Work with Minorities: A European Perspective*, and is currently completing his PhD at Warwick University on the subject of 'Anti-racist Social Work and Postmodernity'.

Neil Thompson, Ph.D. is a Director of Avenue Consulting Ltd (www.avenue consulting.co.uk) and is Visiting Professor in Social Work at the University of Liverpool. He has worked with many organisations in addressing diversity and discrimination issues and is the author of *Anti-Discriminatory Practice* (2001, Palgrave) now in its third edition.

Dylan Ronald Tomlinson, Ph.D. is an Educational Consultant. His current interests are in personal and staff development and he undertakes research in a range of health and social services contexts. He is joint editor, with Kevin Allen, of *Crisis Services and Hospital Crises* (1999, Ashgate Publishing).

Winstow Trew is Co-Director, with Dylan Tomlinson, of T & T Consultants (www.tandtconsultants.co.uk) and his current research interests are in urban regeneration, capacity building and social inclusion. He has extensive experience as a course director, trainer and educator, gained in a variety of higher education settings, where he has specialised in teaching social theory and policy studies.

Jan Wallcraft is a Research Associate at the Sainsbury Centre for Mental Health Services Development and is a user/survivor of psychiatric services. She is a long-time campaigner for, and writer on, alternatives to psychiatric hospital treatment, is a contributor to *Asylum in the Community* (1996, Routledge), and is undertaking a Ph.D. on users' experience of crises.

Acknowledgements

Thanks to Mohan Luthra, of the National Institute for Ethnic Studies in Health and Social Policy (NIESH), and to Waqar Ahmad, of the University of Leeds, who kindly chaired debates on anti-discriminatory practice that the editors organised during 1999 and 2000. Thanks also to Geoffrey Mercer of the University of Leeds for his patient help in facilitating the meetings at which these debates took place.

Introduction

This book is about the strategies that have been devised to counter unfair discrimination in health and social services against women, older people, minority ethnic groups and disabled people. It reviews the development of these strategies in the period since the late 1980s and offers a critical appreciation of proposals for their further implementation in the early years of the twenty-first century.

It is important to recognise that anti-discriminatory strategies are very varied in their nature and in their implications. On the one hand, there are the more conventional and perhaps more widely acceptable strategies which seek to impose a scrupulous degree of fairness in relation to both employment matters and to the provision of services. Foci of such strategies are generally on 'access' issues and 'entry gates'. On the other hand, there are less conventional strategies which seek to mitigate entrenched levels of disadvantage experienced by particular groups, and in some cases to redress the imbalances of employment and services that have resulted from the pattern of disadvantage. These latter strategies have a focus on changing the core values of service 'cultures', so that they reflect the world views of the disadvantaged groups at least as much as those of the advantaged.

While equality of opportunity has long been established as a fairly uncontentious shibboleth of contemporary liberalism, anti-discrimination is more controversial as a concept. This is evident both in successive governments' preference for the term 'non-discrimination', and in the fact that the 'take-up' of both concept and approach has been largely within the social services context, though there are now some signs of its dissemination in the health service, a process in which the editors have had some interest. Ironically, as Dylan Tomlinson indicates in Chapter 1, anti-discrimination was the term used to describe successive bills to outlaw discrimination against racial minorities and against women presented to Parliament in the period before the Race Relations and Sex Discrimination Acts were passed, and these proposals were then accepted by the governments of the day. Thus the phrase 'anti-discrimination' was wholly respectable at that time.

2 Dylan Ronald Tomlinson and Winston Trew

During the early 1990s, anti-racist practice, which had been developed under the auspices of the then Central Council for Education and Training in Social Work (CCETSW), came under prolonged attack from a variety of quarters. This episode is vividly recounted in the form of Naina Patel's 'story' in Chapter 2 which also points to parallels with contemporary attacks on immigrants. The debate about the advantages and disadvantages of anti-racism in social work and welfare from that period, which has run on into discussion of the anti-discriminatory and anti-oppressive practice strategies subsequently developed, has provided a significant stimulus for this book. During the two years preceding its publication, the editors organised a number of meetings to provide an opportunity for debate of these issues. Singh's chapter sets out the key political issues that underpin these debates and draws attention to the way in which anti-racist and anti-oppressive practice are often perceived as inherently threatening, particularly as a challenge to the widespread belief in the fairness and tolerance of British, and by implication the National Health Service (NHS) and Social Services culture.

The attacks on CCETSW's anti-racism were, as Patel and Dominelli's work has shown and as they eloquently discuss in Chapters 2 and 4, inaccurate, misplaced and damaging to social welfare, as well as constituting gratuitous and inflammatory interventions in the general social policy field. Nonetheless there were significant and still unresolved problems with anti-racism and subsequent anti-discriminatory approaches, which were drawn out within the informed discussions of social scientists, health and welfare academics and the professions at the time, and these form a principal concern of the editors. As Winston Trew's discussion demonstrates in the concluding chapter, the major difficulty is that anti-discriminatory approaches continue to reproduce and reinforce – unwittingly in significant, yet little analysed respects – the identification of boundary lines around marginalised groups and their 'problem' status. Lena Dominelli's chapter assesses the impact of particular postmodernist approaches in this regard. She suggests, in setting out the contours of an anti-oppressive practice which takes these approaches into account, that the self needs to be seen as multifaceted and multi-dimensional and that attention needs to be given to the interactive process of identity formation.

Within the health service, approaches to discrimination tend to have been subsumed within well worn equal opportunities policies, but with little priority given to implementation issues or to monitoring taking place to determine how far policy has been put into action. We hope, in this book, that the frameworks set out by Neuberger and Coker, in Chapter 6 and by Uduak Archibong in Chapter 7, go some considerable way toward setting out the scope for change in these respects in the NHS.

The book provides two chapters relating to disability, which it would be fair to say has been of minor rather than major note in the concerns of anti-discrimination. Geoffrey Mercer explores commonalities and discontinuities between the objectives of disabled people's campaigns against discrimination and the emergence of anti-oppressive practice. Jan Wallcraft's chapter provides an illustration of projects nurtured in the voluntary sector which have successfully countered exclusion from work by means of strategies ranging from collective 'self provisioning' to supported transitions to paid employment.

It could be argued that 'equalising oppression, minimising opportunities' would be a more accurate way of describing the pattern of health and welfare services during the period of retrenchment that is generally agreed to have characterised the UK in the 1980s and 1990s. Equality of opportunity does of course have the implication that, in order for individual progression to occur, opportunity has to be parcelled out, and there will be many who are not able to take opportunities or who are judged not able to benefit from them in education or employment contexts. Those who do progress will inevitably, in the fullness of time, be occupants of positions in which they are exerting authority over those who do not. Given that authority is often experienced as over-bearing, especially in a context where individual productivity – getting the most out of the worker – is the lot of the supervisor, the manager, the 'progressor', then maximal oppression can easily be seen as the comfortable counterpart of equality of opportunity. As Neil Thompson discusses in Chapter 3 in the course of outlining his influential approach to anti-discriminatory practice, there are many pitfalls awaiting those who embark on this practice strategy and these must always be considered within their political and social context. Achieving change of this kind is a long-term task whose difficulty should not, he suggests, be underestimated and in which rhetoric and conceptual mazes can easily frustrate the best laid plans.

Finally, it should be noted that, as editors, we have not of course asked contributors to 'sign up' to a particular anti-discriminatory mandate, and there are a number of salient points of disagreement and 'lack of fit' between the various approaches and between our critical appreciations and those approaches. We offer these as a virtue of the book and a stimulus to the eternal task of an informed questioning of theory and practice which has the goal of their enhancement in view.

Chapter I

From equal opportunities to anti-oppressive practice

The historical and social context

Dylan Ronald Tomlinson

This chapter briefly examines the background to the development of equal opportunities and anti-discrimination in health and welfare, beginning with a consideration of some of the early usage of these terms in a civil rights context, then moving on to discuss how interest in anti-discrimination first manifested itself in social work. The concluding section describes the principal features of each of the main approaches to anti-discriminatory practice that have evolved. In focusing on the way in which the civil rights background provided a foundation for anti-discrimination, the chapter is principally concerned with gender and ethnicity.[1]

The origins of UK equal opportunities

Equal opportunities and anti-discrimination are both terms which were commonly used in civil rights struggles in the United States in the mid twentieth century (Cashmore, 1994; Robertson, 1997; Street *et al.*, 1967), although, as Coote and Campbell (1982: 17) suggest 'while women's liberation in Britain drew some considerable inspiration from the United States, it had its own independent beginnings'. These beginnings included women trade unionists setting up an equal pay campaign in the 1950s and taking radical strike action on this issue in high profile disputes during 1968. These disputes culminated in a government commitment to introduce legislation for equal pay. The 'independent beginnings' also included outstanding contributions to the development of socialist feminist thought, one of which (Rowbotham, 1969) is argued to have had 'a profound influence on the development of feminism'.

Although a Royal Commission on Equal Pay was instituted in 1944, its role was limited to evaluating the likely effects of introducing equal pay for equal work and it was not asked to make recommendations. The Commission 'gave little encouragement to the broad application of equal pay' (Office of Manpower Economics, 1972), finding that in most areas outside public service, the work undertaken by men and women was different.

Evans (1944) describes the proposal for an Equal Citizenship (Blanket) Bill to abolish discrimination against women in all its social and economic aspects, from lunacy at one end of the spectrum to employment at the other. She recounts how the hopes of women's organisations for more democracy were dashed during the Second World War. Quite the opposite to the desired process of reform was held to have taken place with 'a wide range of laws, orders and regulations introduced since the outbreak of armed hostilities [continuing] to embody in one form or another some of the worst features of traditional and customary sex discriminations against women' (p. 3). As a consequence of this situation the Women's Publicity Planning Association set up two inquiries in relation to what they argued was anti-democratic practice. The first was an investigation into Acts of Parliament which contained sex discrimination. The second was an investigation into the instances of discrimination freshly introduced by the actions and policies of public or semi-public bodies in the period since war had been declared.

Evans' view is of course consistent with the often pilloried attribution by Beveridge of the breadwinner role to the male head of household (LWLC, 1979). Her emphasis on the need for more democracy to address discrimination against women was part of a broader conception of equal opportunity that links it to the later evolution of 'catch all' organisational policies prescribing equal treatment for a range of social groups commonly subject to discrimination, particularly ethnic minorities and disabled people, in addition to women. Thus Hughes (1968: 40) contends that 'at least since 1944 the British nation has been committed, as a major social priority, to the establishment of a democratic education system which would provide equality of educational opportunity according to "age, ability and aptitude"'. By the 1960s, Hughes' comments on education suggest, equal opportunities were as much associated with countering 'positive discrimination in favour of the middle class' and with establishing 'positive discrimination in favour of deprived areas', as with the position of women in society.

Snell et al. (1981: 2) suggest that up to 1970 equal pay, rather than equal opportunity, was the priority for women's organisations. Two particular pressures, in their view, led to the equal pay movement gaining momentum during the 1950s and 1960s. The first was a shift in position within the TUC, which had hitherto seen voluntary collective bargaining as the means to achieve parity and which, in 1961, recognised that legislation might be a necessary expedient by calling for the government to ratify the International Labour Organisation (ILO) Convention on Equal Pay. The second source of pressure arose from the contingency of the UK wishing to join the EEC, since the Treaty of Rome obliged member countries to make legislative provision to secure 'equal remuneration for the same work' (ibid: 3).

In 1970, an Equal Pay Act was finally passed. As Snell and her colleagues (1981: 2) point out, when the Act received assent in 1970 it was exactly 82 years after an 1888 TUC resolution calling for 'equal pay for the same work', thus constituting 'the longest standing wage claim in the history of the trade union movement'.

By 1969, Coote and Campbell (1982: 15) note that a few women's groups had been set up in Britain, with most of those belonging to such groups being 'members of the left wing intelligentsia – a staunchly masculine society in which women were active and committed, yet felt themselves confined to the periphery'. In February 1970 the first National Women's Liberation Conference was held at Ruskin College, Oxford, an event which had evolved, by chance, from women's dissatisfaction with history workshops at the College proceeding 'as though the female sex had no part in history at all' (ibid.: 20). Among other matters discussed, such as campaigning for free contraception and abortion on demand, were proposals to lobby for a Sex Discrimination Act.

In each year between 1967 and 1973, bills were introduced into the House of Commons to make discrimination against women illegal. The 1972 'Anti-discrimination (no. 2) Bill' for example, had as its objective to 'make illegal and provide for the prevention of discrimination on grounds of sex'. Toward this objective the bill proposed the setting up of an Anti-discrimination Board. The Board was to secure a settlement of differences in case of discrimination and 'an assurance against further discrimination by any party against whom a complaint is proved'. This was the second of two bills introduced by Labour members of the House of Commons in 1972, both of which attracted considerable support within the women's movement. As a consequence of Select Committee reports on the anti-discrimination issues raised by these bills, in both Houses of Parliament, a White Paper was finally published by the Conservative government in September 1973 (Department of Employment, 1973).

The White Paper was titled 'Equal Opportunities for Men and Women' and perhaps with some significance, as will be discussed further below, the government of the day preferred to see its proposals as directed against 'unfair discrimination' and as having the objective of ensuring 'non-discrimination'. Subsequent to the White Paper, the Sex Discrimination Act was passed in 1975. With the Equal Opportunities Commission (EOC) being set up by the Act wholly for the purpose of addressing discrimination against women, gender was formally signified, at least in relation to UK law and politics, as the primary domain for application of the concept of equal opportunities.

Coote and Campbell (1982) record how the omissions in the scope of the government planned legislation, such as pensions, taxation and social security, attracted significant protest within the women's movement, and that the proposed Sex Discrimination Bill was described by one group, in 1973, as consisting of only a 'limited equal opportunities Bill'. They go on to suggest that at least some of the 'feeble effect' of the 1970s' legislation can be attributed to these major deficiences.

The Sex Discrimination Act did, however, possess some features which could be regarded as 'enlightened' for the time. An important feature of the way in which the Equal Opportunities Commission was set up was the lesson learned by government from weaknesses in the functions of the Race Relation Board, as the latter was constructed under the 1965 and 1968 Race Relation Acts; these weaknesses were addressed in the 1976 Act through the establishment of the Commission for Racial Equality (EOC, 1976; Runnymede Trust, 1979). One problem had been that the Board's agenda was complaint led: it could not initiate its own programme of priority issues for investigation or determine particular organisations whose policies merited inspection. In consequence of this problem, the Sex Discrimination Act provided for individuals to take cases to industrial tribunals and County Courts, thus allowing the EOC to concentrate on the wider picture of discrimination in the areas under the Act. A related problem had been that many potential complainants did not come forward because they had good reasons to expect the failure of their case. For that reason the EOC was given powers of its own accord to investigate situations where it believed there might be discrimination, and without the necessity of initiation by those subject to discrimination.

The National Health Service

Equal opportunities policies were slow to develop in the NHS, and indeed it was not required by the Sex Discrimination Act to adopt such policies. Davies and Rosser's (1986) research found that there was a climate of hostility towards equal opportunities policies with regard to women, in the sense that the male career path in which the employee was one hundred per cent committed to work, was regarded as the norm, with women's family commitments leading to support for the widespread assumption that they were rarely in a position to meet that commitment requirement. 'In particular . . . rarely did anyone feel it was justified to take measures to aid women with domestic commitments to take a full part in the organisation. There seemed no financial logic to providing nurseries or any other form of child care, and the moral logic of special training initiatives for women was regarded as dubious' (p. 30).

While it was the case that, by 1982, a number of health authorities advertised themselves as 'equal opportunity employers', Davies and Rosser could find no health authority which had adopted an equal opportunity programme and made arrangements for its monitoring and evaluation (p. 14).

By the mid 1990s, however, the NHS Executive had established an Equal Opportunity Unit, designed to draw together health service initiatives in race, disability and gender, and the Executive asserted that 'as one of the largest employers in Europe the NHS is committed to becoming an equal opportunity employer' (NHS Executive, 1996).

Nonetheless, as Archibong discusses in Chapter 7 of this volume, the problem remains in many NHS Trusts one of monitoring the impact of equal opportunities policies both in relation to data on recruitment and retention of staff and in relation to staff's own views of the usefulness of the policies.

During a 1999 national visit to units providing services to catchment areas with significant black and ethnic minority populations, the Mental Health Act Commission (Warner *et al.*, 2000) found that 23 out of 104 units had developed 'policies procedures or guidelines on training in race equality and anti-discriminatory practice for staff', indicating some degree of NHS engagement with this area of work.

The Commission's use of the term anti-discriminatory practice, though, was informed by the input to the visit of specialist academic researchers. Equal opportunities remains the government's preferred conceptual framework for addressing discrimination in the NHS against both women and minority ethnic groups – as it was in 1973. *The Vital Connection* (NHS Executive, 1999), for example, a strategy for both human resources in the NHS and the deployment of the service in 'local partnership action for community renewal, tackling social exclusion and health inequalities', has a focus on 'equality', 'fair treatment', 'equality of opportunity', 'fair access', and 'fair outcomes'.

The origins of UK anti-discrimination in terms of 'race'

Kushnick (1971) distinguishes the negative concerns of UK politicians with immigration control, culminating in the Commonwealth Immigrants Act of 1962, from the growth, in the mid 1960s, 'mainly from the Labour Party, but also from some Conservatives', of interest in what he calls more positive government activity, including anti-discrimination legislation. Kushnick dates the origins of British efforts at anti-discrimination activity to 1950, when Sorenson introduced a bill to make discrimination in public places a criminal offence. Sorenson's efforts were followed by those of Brockway, starting in 1956, when he introduced the first of nine unsuccessful bills to make discrimination in public houses, lodging houses and dance halls a criminal offence, and, in addition, to criminalise acts of discrimination in the hiring and firing of employees by all employers of more than fifty people. These bills were significant, Kusknick points out, in that Harold Wilson, for the Labour Opposition, twice promised, during 1963 – once in a House of Commons debate and once in a public meeting – that if Parliament continued to reject the Brockway bills, then when there was a Labour majority in the House of Commons the measure would be enacted.

Solomos (1989) suggests that throughout the period from 1945 to 1962 an increasingly racialised debate about immigration took place, focusing on the supposed social problems of having too many black migrants and the question of how they could be stopped from entering given their legal rights under the 1948 British Nationality Act. As Bourne (1980: 332) points out, even in the early UK studies of black immigrant communities – such as those of Kenneth Little (1948), Anthony Richmond (1954) and Michael Banton (1959) which took place in the locations where black settlement long preceded the Second World War: those of Cardiff, Liverpool and London's East End respectively – the focus was on how far cultural assimilation of the 'stranger' was taking place, 'almost as if white hostility was an inevitable and understandable part of human nature'.

Solomos dates the history of anti-discrimination policies in Britain back somewhat later than Kushnick, to the early 1960s,

> when first the Conservative governments of 1958–1964, and then the Labour governments of 1964–1970, developed a view of race and immigration which combined acceptance of the demands for controls on immigration with the proclamation that those migrants already resident should be protected from discrimination and benefit from government action to give them 'equality of opportunity' with their white counterparts.
>
> (Solomos, 1989: 35)

The Race Relations Act 1965 made it unlawful to discriminate on the grounds of colour, race or ethnic or national origins to those seeking access to services and facilities in public places. These public places included hotels, restaurants, theatres, cinemas, public transport and dance halls. The Crown was exempt, though not statutory services such as those provided by the NHS. A Race Relations Board was established to secure compliance with the Act and to initiate investigations, to arbitrate and to establish local conciliation committees for this purpose, and where arbitration failed, or where there appeared to be a lack of compliance with an agreement not to discriminate, to refer clear cases of discrimination to the Attorney General for the purpose of his considering possible prosecution.

The hypocrisy of juxtaposing measures for the control of immigration with this anti-discrimination measure can be seen to have induced, to a degree, a crisis of conscience in the Labour Party. Roy Hattersley, then a Parliamentary Secretary in the Ministry of Labour and MP for Sparkbrook, Birmingham, recalls that the 1968 Commonwealth Immigration Bill, rushed through the House of Commons by a Labour government

had one purpose: to prevent East African Asians coming to Britain. . . .
I had no doubt that Britain had more than a moral obligation to
welcome the refugees to the mother country. We had promised them
refuge at the time of East African independence. The bill broke that
promise. On every night of the extended Committee stage, Shirley
Williams (then Minister of State at the Department of Education) and
I agonised about whether we should go or stay (in the government).
We took the wrong decision.

(Hattersley, 1995: 64)

Ginsburg (1992: 160) argues that there were three factors which prompted
Labour and Conservative governments to implement increasingly restrictive
immigration and nationality laws which differentially affected black people
from the former colonies. These were: first, the overt racist pressures of the
1950s riots; second, Powellism in the late 1960s; and third, the rise to promi-
nence of the National Front in the 1970s. In terms of the first of Ginsburg's
three factors, Williams (1987) suggests that the racism of the Notting Hill
riots can be accounted for by the 'historical concessions to racialist and
racist ideology' made by the white working class, and by the fear within
that class that the welfare state was 'shortchanging' it, particularly in relation
to housing. In terms of the second of Ginsburg's factors, as Sondhi (1994: 38)
points out, the community action initiatives which were developed as part
of the 'positive' response to imigration, under Section 11 of the 1966 Local
Government Act, however well intentioned, were set against a context of
'sustained hostility towards black people, issuing from all sections of a
class society and many of its major institutions'. This context, Sondhi
suggests, led to the development of ethnically self-conscious radical group-
ings which became inevitably disaffected from municipal politics and
welfare.

In 1967, Street et al., as 'experts' in the field, were asked by the UK government to examine the anti-discrimination laws of other countries with a view
to modifying UK law. The 'Street' Committee looked in particular at both
the Federal and State laws of the USA and at Canadian laws. An interesting
feature of the report (1967) that Street and his colleagues produced is the
description of the pressure for national law which was applied by black
people in the USA during the Second World War. Although the policy of
the Federal government in the 1940s was one of non-discrimination, there
was widespread discrimination in the defence industries, and, as a consequence, a march on Washington, which was predicted to be likely to
number over 100,000 was called by black leaders. As Street comments,
'in war-time a protest on this scale could not be ignored'. The President
promised action and the march was called off. So was initiated Executive
Order 8802, which reaffirmed that there should be no discrimination in the
employment of workers in defence industries or government, on the grounds

of race, colour or national origin, with the order providing further for 'the full and equitable participation of all workers in defence industries, without discrimination'. A President's Committee on Fair Employment Practice was set up to investigate complaints of discrimination and although the Committee had no specific powers, it was able to achieve, according to Street, some compliance with its directives.

The Street Report is an important document in so far as it established that the origins of anti-discrimination legislation can be fairly clearly traced to the Ives-Quinn Act of 1945, which prohibited racial discrimination, and, following the precedent of the President's Commission, established a New York State Commission Against Discrimination. As well as having the duty to arbitrate, this Commission had recourse to legal sanction and was able to call a public hearing and issue orders requiring respondents to desist from discrimination and to order the payment of compensatory damages to the complainant. The New York model was followed in most states in the period up to the Civil Rights Act of 1964.

The Street Report was one of two interrelated Political and Economic Planning reports. The other report, 'Racial Discrimination' published in the same year, indicated widespread discrimination in the UK in employment, housing, insurance, credit facilities and financial services. According to Kushnick (1971: 253), although the report's findings provided no surprises for those concerned with the issues, 'they did have a dramatic impact on the mass media and on public opinion' and 'newspaper leaders gave an overwhelming degree of support for new legislation'.

What were the forms of resistance to equal opportunities and anti-discrimination legislation?

Both Street and Kushnick point to the obstructiveness of trade unions, in a number of instances, in the USA and in the UK respectively, with regard to the implementation of anti-racial discrimination law in the period after the Second World War. While the Equal Opportunities Commission (1976: 6) on one hand, noted 'a variety of obstacles to equal opportunity', many of which were described as being based on taken-for-granted assumptions and 'stereotypes', the Commission was also 'acutely aware . . . of the strong under-current of resentment [by employers] against . . . an excessive and growing burden of legislation'. In addition to the Equal Pay Act – implemented over the period from 1970 to 1975 – and the Sex Discrimination Act, there were also the Employment Protection Act, The Trade Union and Labour Relations Act, the Race Relations Act, and the Health and Safety at Work Act. It had, the Commission went on to record, 'been difficult in these circumstances to persuade employers that the Sex Discrimination Act and the Equal Pay Act' were 'not just merely two pieces of legislation with which they have to comply' but were 'of direct relevance to their whole range of policies and practices'.

Why social work as anti-discrimination?

This is a difficult question to answer. Part of the answer perhaps lies in the impact of the political and intellectual libertarianism of the late 1960s and 1970s on those with a vocational commitment to the welfare of people suffering extreme social disadvantage. As Sondhi (1994: 37–8) comments, the rise of 'single issue' campaigns concerned with world hunger, colonial freedom, nuclear disarmament, child poverty, homelessness and racial equality provided a 'refreshing change from the tired and predictable styles of all brands of left wing socialism'. In Britain in the late sixties these campaigns, many of which, of course, occupied the central ground of social work, 'found resonance in and picked up momentum from the cataclysmic events happening elsewhere in the world – the student revolutions in Europe, the growing protests against the Vietnam war, the rise of the black struggle and of black power in the United States'.

Partly, too, the rise of anti-discriminatory practice in social work can be attributed to its location, educationally, within social policy and administration. An indication of the 'rupture' in the main streams of socialist and feminist analyses in this area can be found in the debates of the *Critical Social Policy* editorial collective. This 'socialist and feminist welfare journal', founded in 1981, publicly aired conflict between its black and white collective members in 1987. The three black members stated that they had 'provisionally withdrawn their participation until such time that key issues on race, racism and anti-racism have been seriously acknowledged and dealt with by our white colleagues'. The statement went on to say that although the three black members had not met each other before the December 1986 meeting of the collective 'it would appear that we were immediately united by our common experience of having to cope with racism – even in its most liberal guises'. Continuing by pointing to the lack of support from white members in the struggle of the then one black member of the collective, over the course of a year, to have racism issues seriously addressed, the statement pointed out that 'the problems and contradictions within the *CSP* collective appear to be typical of the difficulty which the white left have in coming to a realistic understanding of racism and their involvement in it'. 'Anti-racism', the statement continued, 'is not simply about getting some blacks to join the Collective, important as it is . . . it is about interrogating the underlying premises of much of the knowledge produced in the metropolitan societies, *not merely bourgeois knowledge but also socialist and feminist theory*' (emphasis added).

The white members of the collective responded with a statement of principle in which they recognised that 'the responsibility for racism and our attitude towards it as white members of the Collective lies with us and there is a responsibility for us to advance that understanding and our practice'. Further, the white members stated that the criteria for publication 'should include an awareness of racism and anti-racist struggles and experiences, and of current debates and thinking about the relationship between racism and (in particular) class and gender oppression'.

Day (1992) suggests that the women's movement had generally, until the 1980s, been one which, in the interests of unity against sexism, tended to disregard class and race differences in women's experience. The focus on equal rights in political and cultural institutions, and equal rights in employment, meant that issues like 'double shifting' – the hardship of undertaking low paid work outside the home and domestic work inside it rather than being defined by the label 'housewife' – and of cultural and ethnic stereotyping, in the form, for instance, of widespread racist assumptions concerning black women's sexuality and black people's lesser intellectual ability – were downplayed. Nor did radical feminism offer a solution to these issues, since it was, to a significant extent, an array of eurocentric or colonial values rather than patriarchy as such, which dominated their agenda.

The development of anti-discriminatory practice

In this section I review some of the more widely circulated and quoted texts that have been produced in the area of anti-discriminatory practice. However, it does not claim to be comprehensive, either in terms of the output of the writers concerned, or in terms of the range of texts in the field.

Anti-racist social work

Dominelli's iteration of anti-racist social work (Dominelli, 1988) first makes a clear distinction between the development of this form of practice and the pursuit of equal opportunities, and second highlights the detrimental impact on clients, referred to earlier in this chapter, of the process whereby controls on immigration have been held to be justifiable provided that legislation is in place to protect migrants already settled in the UK from discrimination. Third the approach illustrates the mutually reinforcing effects of, on one hand, racism against those she defines as 'non-Anglo-Saxon people', within the social and political structure, and, on the other, the exclusion of minority ethnic groups from services.

In relation to the first point, it is argued that while an equal opportunities policy does create a more helpful climate by providing an organisational context in which minority workers are encouraged to apply for positions and service users to put forward their requirements, it does not mean the transformation of the organisation itself, which is what anti-racist social work would signify.

In relation to the second point, Dominelli argues that the Race Relations Act 'does not merit the label "anti-racist"' (p. 27). She suggests that, because of the environment created by Nationality Acts, which accord respectability to the view that immigrants should have a reduced status, black people become, in effect, the undeserving poor, in contrast to white people as the deserving.

She makes the third point in the following way:

> I take the view that racism aimed specifically at non-Anglo-Saxon people forms part of a larger process of social control. Thus it reinforces the controlling dimension of social work and intensifies the policing aspect of white social workers' relationships with ethnic minority groups and contributes to their exclusion from the creation and delivery of services relevant to their welfare.
>
> (Dominelli, 1988: 17)

Anti-racist social work is then outlined as comprising five elements:

- the development of egalitarian relationships;
- an appreciation of the nature of the process by which the allocation of wealth in society has distinct discriminatory outcomes;
- a shift in the values of the educational curriculum toward the core values of anti-discriminatory practice;
- recognition of the importance of the 'consciousness raising' role of practitioners in anti-racist social work, particularly among their colleagues and in their organisational networks; and
- a politically committed form of practice.

The development of egalitarian relationships

This has several components but the first is for social workers to become aware of the nature of the prejudices which, on account of the kinds of mutual reinforcement noted above, will inevitably have a significant impact on their practice:

> By understanding themselves, their value system, prejudices, position in society and the privileges accruing to them through racist social relations, white social workers can become racially aware in a manner which incorporates both the structural and the personal components of racism, raises their political consciousness of racial issues and rids them personally of racial prejudice, whether intended or not.
>
> (Dominelli, 1988: 73)

Though the processes whereby egalitarian relationships between black clients and white workers are envisaged as being difficult to develop, white people advocating anti-racist social work are held to have a major role in redefining social work to conform to anti-racism. The initial lack of familiarity in working within egalitarian relationships and the corollary of an unfamiliar loss of power over others will, Dominelli suggests:

> initially disorient and overwhelm white social work educators and practitioners . . . an acute awareness of our loss of power and privileges in the short term will obscure the long-term advantages accruing from the anti-racist stance.
>
> (Ibid.: 15)

Society has to change as well as social work, she argues, if this process is to be able to attract support, in the sense that equal opportunities has to be regarded as legitimate rather than a politically motivated redistribution from white working-class to black working-class people.

The second component of building egalitarian relationships is for social workers to build on the self awareness that they can gain through anti-racism, of the impact of prejudice and power, so as to be able to take part in wider organisational change and political action to counter racism. Dominelli urges the following:

> Bearing in mind that the forms racism assumes and our understanding of the steps necessary for its elimination vary over time as socio-econominc conditions change, white social workers can become involved in the struggle to eradicate racism by: a) becoming racially aware individuals; b) working to eliminate institutionalised racism in their agency and in their practice; and c) taking up the anti-racist struggle more generally through political activity.
>
> (Ibid.: 82)

This form of socio-political practice is aimed at having the result that egalitarian relationships, in relation to ethnicity, will at least be characterised by:

- social workers being ethnically sensitive to the different meanings attached to social interaction by people from non-white majority cultures;
- social workers being aware of the cultural diversity within the majority white culture;
- social workers being able to address the boundaries of resource constraints which constrain the making of choices between themselves and clients.

(Ibid.: 32)

An appreciation of the nature of the process by which the allocation of wealth in society has distinct discriminatory outcomes

In Dominelli's view, it is crucial that connections are made by social workers between two social processes that are often presented as quite distinct from each other. On one hand, it is important to take note of the following factors: the draining of resources from welfare in the form of innumerable attempts to redistribute the social security budget among the poor, with minimal augmentation in its value; the restrictions on spending in education, health and social services; the emphases of contemporary governments on law and order and defence; and the general tendency of such governments to concentrate on tax relief for those who are on middle and higher incomes. On the other hand, it is critical for social workers to connect these processes to the representation of black people in the media and in public discourse as overdependent on welfare, indolent and as having a problem status based on such factors as work-attitude.

A shift in the values of the educational curriculum toward the core values of anti-discriminatory practice

Dominelli regards such a change as one that is wholly consistent with well established social work principles:

> shifting the social work curriculum's political bias away from favouring the status quo towards one securing justice for oppressed groups will accord priority to social work's traditional caring values rather than its controlling ones.
>
> (Ibid.: 60)

A major task in combating racism is, for Dominelli, the production of 'theories of welfare which acknowledge social work's social control function; recognise its dual position within state structures – a controller of substantial resources and upholder of a caring ideology; and promote anti-racist social work practice' (p. 35). To do this, it is argued, the social work profession has to adopt a political stance, using its organisations, such as the National Association of Probation Officers and the National Association of Local Government Officers, for this purpose. This involves the profession taking a stance against so-called 'colour blind' views that white and black people should be treated in the same way as each other, and that all human beings are equal, i.e. universalistic approaches that prescribe the same service and the same conditions of entry for all, resulting, for example, in racism in housing by means of length of local residence criteria.

Recognition of the importance of the 'consciousness raising' role of practitioners in anti-racist social work, particularly among colleagues and in organisational networks

'White social workers adopting an anti-racist position have a consciousness-raising role in making white people perceive racism as a social issue', Dominelli (ibid.: 40) suggests, going on to add, in a later section that:

> it is not enough for white social workers developing anti-racist practice to rely on their personal commitment to see them through to successful anti-racist intervention in a black family. White social workers wishing to develop anti-racist social work practice have no option but to initiate the organisational process of changing the perceptions, commitments and behaviour of colleagues, managers, employers and clients in this direction. Employers would have to commit themselves to introducing anti-racist policies and practices in their agency, thus providing the climate and backup support necessary for promoting racial equality and anti-racist social work.
>
> (Ibid.: 123–4)

A politically committed form of practice

This principle means that the profession should, in Dominelli's view, abandon the pretence of objectivity and that it should state its credentials as an 'equalising' profession – i.e. one which is in favour of redistribution from the wealthy to the poor, from men to women and from white to black, so that it is not represented as about depriving one set of poor white clients to give to another set. The profession should give high priority to political action both within organisations and outside organisations, e.g. in immigration campaigns; and it should erase the dividing lines betweeen itself and probation, social security and housing work, thus giving due regard to the shared nature of care tasks across these areas, and so that it can support users to define the kind of services which they wish to receive.

Dominelli illustrates anti-racist social work practice by means of several case studies. It is useful to briefly outline one of the case studies in order to document Dominelli's analysis of the kind of facets of practice which require to be changed if anti-racism is to be taken up.

Case study

A Health Visitor referred a Sikh woman, 'Indejit', who spoke Punjabi but very little English, to social services because she was suffering from post-natal depression after giving birth to a girl. There were no Punjabi speaking black workers in the team so a white worker carried out a home visit. In the home, the eldest daughter, aged nine, acted as interpreter. The worker believed that Indejit was feeling 'down' because she had given birth to four successive daughters. However, she also assessed Indejit as being lonely and so asked a voluntary worker to befriend her and help her learn English. The voluntary agency did not have any black Punjabi speaking workers either but to demonstrate its commitment sent its best worker. The worker noted the relationship between herself and the client to be good and although her depression was not getting better, the worker was aware that the client was seeing her GP and taking prescribed drugs, so she did not raise the subject. When this worker left the agency and another took over it was discovered, by chance, that Indejit had been physically abused on a regular basis by her husband. However, the worker felt there was nothing to be done in the face of this situation, since there was no women's refuge in the town, and no refuge facility for Asian women.

(Adapted from Dominelli, 1988: 102–3)

Dominelli comments that 'this case is obviously one in which collusion with institutionalised racism and sexism is occurring on a massive scale' (p. 103). Social services were not taking responsibility as care agency in that they had no Punjabi speaking black workers, and had not made any inter-agency arrangements to deploy such workers, who could make an adequate assessment of need. No other agency had been set up to address the needs of black clients. The voluntary agency was colluding with racism in taking on the case while knowingly not having the capacity to address its demands. Social workers were going along with racism in undertaking visits while not able to communicate adequately, and adopting racist stereotypes of Asian women in relation to childbirth. The voluntary workers colluded with racism in not addressing the issue of domestic violence.

Anti-racist social work in this instance, Dominelli's account suggests, would require:

• that the social services department made links with others who do have Punjabi speaking Sikh social workers;

- that, since it serves black communities, it should be employing black workers to serve those communities;
- that white anti-racist social workers should press their departments to adopt this strategy;
- that the department should not automatically use a black child as an interpreter, both because of the issues of interaction between the child and the adult and because it sends a message that interpreting needs are not valid or important enough to warrant a service; and
- that the department should not have fallen back, for misplaced humanitarian reasons, on the voluntary sector to provide generic unfocused help, thus excusing social services from responding to the manifest needs involved.

Feminist, anti-discriminatory, anti-oppressive practice

The Feminist approach

Like Dominelli, Langan and Day (1992) aim to break new ground in terms of contributing significantly to the development of a new form of social work practice. The objective of their work, Langan points out, is to 'identify the essential elements of a feminist, non-oppressive, anti-discriminatory practice for the 1990s' (p. 2). Langan argues that 'the movement towards anti-discriminatory social work really took off from the encounter between feminist and anti-racist women in the 1980s' (ibid.). Thereafter, she suggests, it extended in scope to include analyses of discrimination against women in relation to sexual orientation, disability and age as well as to ethnicity, nationality, culture and religion.

Langan gives a useful sketch of trends in social work leading up to the anti-discriminatory epistemological 'break'. With the creation of the welfare state, and rising levels of prosperity in the decades after the Second World War, the emerging social work profession came to focus on 'problem families' who were not thriving and taking advantage of the favourable social and economic environment. Various psychologically based approaches with an emphasis on maladjustment of families and individuals, were in favour. These approaches came under attack in the 1970s with the advent of radical social work, which, in a then worsening economic climate, highlighted class, poverty, unemployment and other major sources of social inequality as of primary importance in assessing and responding to clients' difficulties. Within this strand of social work, alliances with working-class institutions, such as tenants groups, community associations and trade unions, were advocated as a more effective means of collective social work action than individual casework, which could have little effect on the oppressive structure of clients' situations.

The growth of the women's movement and of the numbers of feminist social workers then produced a re-appraisal of radical social work, which had had little to offer in terms of appreciating the critical issue of the majority of both workers and clients in social services: most were women, and most were subject, in practice, to a male dominated form of professional and organisational control. Demands for a feminist social work that could take account of diversity – in terms of age, disability and ethnicity – built up during the late 1980s (pp. 2–3).

An interesting feature of Langan and Day's (1992) analysis is that, as with anti-racist practice and anti-oppressive practice, engagement with the issues of disability is somewhat marginal. Williams is the sole contributor to the text who addresses this area of practice, and the focus is on learning disability, a form of disability which had not been a salient concern of the disability movement or of disability studies (Walmsley, 2001). A significant theme in Williams' discussion is that of stereotyping and the importance of not colluding with this common form of discrimination. Thus Williams analyses the way in which people with learning disabilities have been endowed with child-like attributes, especially innocence. The traditional views in British social work were bound up with eugenics and poor mothering and the importance of the learning disabled not having children and thus debasing the quality of the national stock. The idea of taking risks and supporting decisions relating to sexual identity had not been given credence within learning disability services.

Anti-discriminatory practice

Thompson's (1977) framework for anti-discriminatory practice is a widely cited approach which provides an account of social discrimination in relation to gender, ethnicity, age and disability, though other sources of discrimination, such as those encountered in respect of religion and sexual identity, are also briefly reviewed. As he outlines the framework in Chapter 3 of this volume, it will not be discussed in depth here. Briefly, Thompson is concerned with setting out the social origins of each type of discrimination, particularly with regard to the power of ideology, and with enumerating principles for practice to be able to address those forms of discrimination. This enumeration emphasises the importance of social workers taking account of all the aspects of discrimination that may affect individual clients, rather than seeing an individual as 'someone from a particular culture' or 'someone who is disabled'. With some caution, Thompson also stresses the importance of the contribution of social work to the processes by which clients nurture and develop 'positive identities' for themselves. These take place within a context of what may often be hostile and negative social imagery of their particular groups being reproduced in politics and the media.

Thompson notes some similarities between radical social work, in its criticism of the power exercised by the state and by statutory social workers, and the objectives of anti-discriminatory practice, the principal difference being the overturning, within the latter, of the excessive reliance on class analysis that had characterised the former. In noting those similarities, he also draws attention to the fact that achieving anti-discriminatory practice is a long-term goal, and one which is beset by innumerable difficulties, some of which are discussed as 'pitfalls' in his chapter.

Anti-oppressive practice

Published in 1995, Dalrymple and Burke's conceptualisation of anti-oppressive practice is the most recently articulated approach of the four that are discussed in this chapter, though of course it should be noted that Dominelli (2001) outlines a further elaboration of this particular form of practice in Chapter 4 of this volume. I would suggest that their approach can be regarded as having five key elements: a process of self discovery; a focus on the dynamics of the worker–client relationship; as a form of practice which takes place on several levels; a focus on constructive use of the law; and a commitment to redemption.

A process of self-discovery

Anti-oppressive practice is presented as a process of self discovery with relation, in particular, to gender and ethnicity. The discovery is in the sense of social workers (mainly women) recalling experiences such as not being taken seriously as women, being overlooked for promotion, for the same reason, and being considered suitable for distinctively 'female' job opportunities. The same process of self discovery applies to white males, who first can come to an understanding of their own role as an oppressor, or carrier of advantage, and second can come to question assumptions about self and others that accord with that vantage point – such as that males take for granted the assumption of leadership, of the right to speak first in a meeting, of the right to a greater share of resources in terms of language and communication skills, to the disadvantage of others. Acknowledging the differing backgrounds of oppressor and oppressed enables those embarking on the process of self discovery, in knowing the dimensions of their own oppression, to understand better the position of others.

Dalrymple and Burke argue as follows:

> Individuals who make the connections between their personal condition and the society in which they exist begin to make changes within themselves, within their families and community and wider social structures. Individuals who become aware of the connection between their personal

condition and the society in which they exist have the means to evaluate their position critically. Through the process of self discovery we are able to name our oppression but equally we can begin to address the causes of our oppression.

(Dalrymple and Burke, 1995: 12)

A focus on the dynamics of the worker–client relationship

Anti-oppressive practice has a primary focus on the worker's relationship with the client. It is about the worker–client relationship, in several senses:

- in allowing the client to define the nature of the problem, to tell a story and in so doing gain credence, self respect, autonomy by being listened to, and by building the presenting problem in good measure themselves;
- in being interactive, negotiation based, consumerist, grass roots and demand led, thus being a process generative of demands and of the shaping of demands, even in circumstances where the client's behaviour may be the subject of monitoring with a view to the imposition of constraints;
- in having the objective of being egalitarian and power sharing (power is defined loosely in terms of psychological, economic, political, or philosophical aspects and anti-oppressive practice then applies to the recognition of power imbalances in all these areas) the working relationship is to be designed to redress the balance of power, to seek equity in worker–client relations, and make available resources and support to clients in pursuit of these aims; and
- by being based on engagement – practice has got to breach class barriers, and it has to be based on a level of trust and respect for different world views.

A form of practice which take place on several levels

Dalrymple and Burke (1995) suggest that anti-opppressive practice takes place on three levels: construct, strategic and material. Work at the construct level relates to how the problems that clients have are conceptualised; at the strategic level to the techniques to be brought into play and plans of action; and at the material level to the political and social environment, which has always to be borne in mind.

A focus on constructive use of the law

The constructive use of legislation applies, for instance, to such areas as those of local authority obligations to care leavers, assessments of those who are vulnerable, the Care Programme Approach and to social workers being prepared to deploy court orders to support partnership with clients, in some cases, rather than to see their use as always controlling.

A commitment to redemption

- In its commitment to the principle, above all else, that something constructive can be done in all worker–client interactions, and that intervention, whether for assessment or for a programme of care or protection should be about redeemable people – in other words all clients are considered to be growing or susceptible to growth, while, at the same time, it is equally important to assume that the social worker has something to offer.

Oppression in this framework is defined as: 'a system of *colliding explosive forces* [original emphasis] which, if they collide randomly, are more likely to be oppressive'. If these forces are 'channelled and controlled however', Dalrymple and Burke argue, 'they can open up new opportunities'. They go on to cite a case in Devon (1995: 57–60) to show how these colliding forces operate, and it is useful in expounding their approach to include the description of the case in this section.

Case study

The study concerns a girl suspected to have been sexually abused by the male partner of the girl's mother, 'Mr L', who was thought to have been abusing children of his partners in subsequent relationships which were begun after he had left the mother concerned in the original case.

In the initial instance of suspected abuse, which followed on from concerns being expressed by the girl's school teacher about her disturbed behaviour, she stated that she had been touched inappropriately by Mr L. A paediatrician confirmed that the girl's condition indicated her genital area had been manipulated, Mr L was arrested and interviewed by police. He denied the allegations and no charges were ever brought against him.

Over the following two and a quarter years, Mr L had three relationships in which he began living with the partners concerned, in the first of which he had a child with the partner. On each of the three occasions social workers advised the women with whom he was living that a case conference would have to be held to consider possible registration of the children living in the household if he continued living there. In the

first two cases Mr L moved out when requested to do so by the women.
In the third case there was some delay and resistance.
    At some point during this process, though it is not stated when, Mr L
sought help from a solicitor to defend himself.

                         (Abridged from Dalrymple and Burke, 1995.
      Detailed sources are given in Dalrymple and Burke, 1995: 57.)

Dalrymple and Burke point out that the social workers had not, at any stage
had any contact with Mr L, no case conference had ever been held and his
name was not on a list of abusers or a child abuse register. Mr L was illiterate
and understood things differently to the social workers. They see this case as
one of colliding forces in terms of the interest of different professionals, the
women, and Mr L.

What could have happened is engagement with Mr L so as to enable the
possibility of him addressing the behaviour giving offence to be discussed,
to enable him to have the possibility of retaining his relationships with his
partners and with his own child, and to minimise the possibility of adversar-
ial conflict. Mr L, they point out, was disempowered and the process was
based on oppressive forces being directed at him, so limiting the potential
for what they refer to as the positive forces within him to be brought out.

Dalrymple and Burke contend that while anti-oppressive practice is:

> about ensuring that people are not oppressed because of the protective
> nature of our [social workers'] role. It is difficult to think about anti-
> oppressive practice when working with someone who we believe may
> well have abused his own power (as male adult). So the practice is
> about helping that person to understand why his action has been seen
> as an abuse of power.

(Dalrymple and Burke, 1995: 60)

A second case reviewed by Dalrymple and Burke is also useful to consider
briefly, in terms of their comments above about social workers' preparedness
to consider court orders as potentially consistent with partnership. The case
concerns a situation in which a residence order for a child was desired by the
family carers involved, but refused by the justices on the basis that an order
should not be made unless it was a better option than not making an order
(ibid.: 61–2). Since the 11 year-old girl had lived with the grandmother for
all but the first six weeks of her life, they did not see adequate grounds.
But in practice, because of the grandmother's need for legal authority to
be able to deal with such things as medical emergencies and authorisation
for school trips, and because the mother's occasionally disturbed behaviour

might lead her to take the child away, while the child wanted security in the care arrangement, an order would have been appropriate and consistent with anti-oppressive practice. For Dalyrmple and Burke, the decision of the justices clearly was not empowering of either the grandmother or the granddaughter.

Finally, it is noteworthy, in outlining this approach, that Dalrymple and Burke (1995) suggest 'it could be argued that the use of the word intervention is oppressive and by its very nature indicates where the power base lies'. They go on to comment that 'given such an observation, perhaps a more useful way of describing the process could be that *interaction* [original emphasis] takes place rather than intervention' (p. 89). However, they qualify this point by saying that this would only be suitable in cases of minimal intervention, as otherwise it might convincingly be argued to be dishonest in cases involving compulsion.

Meanings and implications in the terms used to describe principles of practice which are aimed to counter discrimination

It is ironic that 'anti-discrimination', from being a wholly liberal strategy to safeguard the civil rights of women and minority ethnic groups during the post-Second World War period, came to be both conceptualised and regarded, in a social work context, as a radical challenge to the values of the British welfare state and of British culture. The term 'anti-oppressive' on the other hand can be seen to have rather deeper roots as part of a much analysed 'British' popular radical tradition. In the pre-Chartist late eighteenth-century and early nineteenth-century periods, when the 'Combination Acts' were in force prohibiting popular gatherings concerning trade or political matters (these were construed as usurping the King's authority and potentially seditious), and when spies and informers drove popular radicalism underground, the word oppression held an important place in the demagoguery of the period. The 'people' were constructed as firm in opposition and resistance to the oppression of 'Old Corruption' by which was meant the buying and selling of public offices and titles, (including seats in Parliament); the venal trading of the national interest in aristocratic intrigues designed solely to augment personal fortunes; and impressment, the practice of rounding up men into conscript armies to support those aristocratic intrigues in wars between Britain and its European rivals (Saville, 1954; Thompson, 1968; Joyce, 1995).

As an address to the General Body of Mechanics of 1818 declaimed:

> the broad and malignant grasps of aristocracy, extended out by a cruel and overbearing number of employers, have acted as an opaque body over the sun of your rights and independence – have intercepted all

the cheering rays of social and domestic happiness, leaving you nothing but the winter of poverty and oppression to travel through to your very graves.

(Cited in Aspinall 1949: 311)

Set against this conceptual background, at least, anti-oppressive practice is suggestive of an undoubtedly radical politics.

Note

1 The chapter does not address disability, since its objective is to provide a brief account of the origins of anti-discrimination concepts and connect them to the development of anti-discriminatory practice, rather than to review all influences on the latter. As the work of both Oliver (1990) and Davis (1993) suggests, the disability activism of the late 1980s and 1990s, culminating in the launch of a campaign for anti-discrimination legislation at the British Council of Organisations of Disabled People Annual General Meeting in 1991, was subject to the influence of earlier women's and minority ethnic group's campaigns.

References

Aspinall, A. (1949) *The Early English Trade Unions*, London: Batchworth Press.

Banton, M. (1959) *White and Coloured: The Behaviour of British People Towards Coloured Immigrants*, London: Cape.

Black members of the CSP Collective (1987) 'Statement by the black members of the CSP Collective', *Critical Social Policy*, vol. 7, no. 1.

Bourne, J. (1980) 'Cheerleaders and ombudsmen: the sociology of race relations in Britain', *Race and Class*, vol. 21, no. 4.

Cashmore, E. (1994) *Dictionary of Race and Ethnic Relations*, London: Routledge.

Coote, A. and Campbell, B. (1982) *Sweet Freedom: The Struggle for Women's Liberation*, London: Pan Books.

Dalrymple, J. and Burke, B. (1995) *Anti-Oppressive Practice: Social Care and the Law*, Buckingham: Open University Press.

Davies, C. and Rosser, J. (1986) *Processes of Discrimination: A Study of Women Working in the NHS*, London: DHSS.

Davis, K. (1993) 'On the Movement', in Swain, J., Finkelstein, V., French, S. and Oliver, M. (eds) *Disabling Barriers – Enabling Environments*, London: Sage.

Day, L. (1992), 'Women and oppression: race class and gender', in Langan, M. and Day, L. (eds), *Women, Oppression and Social Work*, London: Routledge.

Department of Employment (1973) *Equal Opportunities for Men and Women: Government Proposals for Legislation*, London: HMSO.

Dominelli, L. (1988) *Anti-Racist Social Work: A Challenge for White Practitioners and Educators*, Basingstoke: Macmillan.

Equal Opportunities Commission (1976) *The Annual Report of the Equal Opportunities Commission 1976*, London: HMSO.

Evans, D. (1944) *Equal Citizenship (Blanket) Bill*, London: Women's Publicity Planning Association.

Ginsburg, N. (1992) *Divisions of Welfare: A Critical Introduction to Comparative Social Policy*, London: Sage.

Hattersley, R. (1995) *Who Goes Home: Scenes from a Political Life*, London: Little, Brown and Company.

Hughes, H. D. (1968) 'How far is selectivity necessary in education?', in Townsend, P., Reddin, M., Kaim-Caudle, P., Hughes, H. D., Davies, B., Harvey, A., Nevitt, D. A., Owen, D. and Abel-Smith, B., *Social Services for All ?* London: Fabian Society.

House of Commons (1972) *Anti-Discrimination (no. 2) Bill*, London: House of Commons.

Joyce, P. (ed.) (1995) *Class*, Oxford: Oxford University Press.

Kushnick, L. (1971) 'British anti-discrimination legislation', in Abbott, S., *The Prevention of Racial Discrimination in Britain*, London: Oxford University Press.

Langan, M. and Day, L. (eds) (1992) *Women, Oppression and Social Work*, London: Routledge.

Little, K. (1947) *Negroes in Britain: A Study of Race Relations in English Society*, London: Kegan Paul.

Little, K. (1956) *The Race Question in Modern Science*, Paris: UNESCO.

London Women's Liberation Campaign for Legal and Financial Independence *and* Rights of Women (LWLC) (1979) 'Disaggregation now', *Feminist Review*, no. 2.

NHS Executive (1996) *Annual Report – 1995/6*, London: NHS Executive.

NHS Executive (1999) *The Vital Connection*, London: Stationery Office.

Office of Manpower Economics (1972) *Equal Pay*, London: HMSO.

Oliver, M. (1990) *The Politics of Disablement*, Basingstoke: Macmillan.

Racial Discrimination (1967) Report of Political and Economic Planning, London: Political and Economic Planning.

Richmond, A.H. (1954) *Colour Prejudice in Britain: A Study of West Indian Workers in Liverpool 1942–1951*, London: Routledge.

Robertson, D. (1997) *A Dictionary of Human Rights*, London: Europa Publications.

Rowbotham, S. (1969) *Women's Liberation and the New Politics*, Spokesman's Pamphlet No. 17, Nottingham: Spokesman].

Runnymede Trust (1979) *A Review of the Race Relations Act 1976*, London: Runnymede Trust.

Saville, J. (ed.) (1954) *Democracy and the Labour Movement: Essays in honour of Dona Torr*, London: Lawrence and Wishart.

Snell, M. W., Glucklich, P. and Povall, M. (1981) *Equal Pay and Opportunities: A Study of the Implementation and Effects of the Equal Pay and Sex Discrimination Acts in 26 Organisations*, London: Department of Employment.

Solomos, J. (1989) *Race and Racism in Contemporary Britain*, Basingstoke: Macmillan.

Sondhi, R. (1994) 'From Black British to Black European: a crisis of identity?', in Jacobs, S. and Popple, K., *Community Work in the 1990s*, Nottingham: Spokesman.

Street, H., Howe, G. and Bindman, G. (1967) *Anti-Discrimination Legislation*, London: Political and Economic Planning.

The Editorial Collective (1987) 'Towards an anti-racist publishing practice', *Critical Social Policy*, vol. 7, no. 1.

Thompson, E. P. (1968) *The Making of the English Working Class*, Harmondsworth: Penguin.

Thompson, N. (1997) *Anti-Discriminatory Practice*, Basingstoke: Macmillan.

Walmsley, J. (2001) 'Normalisation, Emancipatory Research and Inclusive Research in Learning Disability', *Disability and Society*, vol. 16, no. 2.

Warner, L., Nicholas, S., Patel, K., Harris, J. and Ford, R. (2000) *National Visit 2: A Visit by the Mental Health Act Commission to 104 Mental Health and Learning Disability Units in England and Wales*, London: Sainsbury Centre for Mental Health.

Williams, F. (1987) 'Racism and the discipline of social policy: a critique of welfare theory', *Critical Social Policy* vol. 7, no. 2.

Chapter 2

The campaign against anti-racism in social work

Racism where? You see it . . . you don't

Naina Patel

> If you are following the party line you don't have to document anything;
> you can say anything you feel like . . .
> On the other hand if you're critical of received opinion,
> you have to document every phrase.
>
> (N. Chomsky 1992 in *Chronicles of Dissent*, AK Press)

Prologue

It is always Sundays *She* thought when the rain breaks, snow falls, stories break. Events happen. After all 'time' is on people's side – Sunday a day of rest – of sorts. And some stories continue, only punctuated by time. The East Yorkshire Conservative MP John Townend claimed that immigrants (*She* thought, yes, he's talking of 'me') were undermining Britain's 'homogeneous Anglo-Saxon society'. Robin Cook the foreign secretary said the Conservative leader, Mr Hague's recent comment that Britain would turn into a 'foreign land' with Labour's second term was just the type of comment that fuelled racist views. In West Yorkshire in Bradford around the same time, the TV screens told of 'mixed race' people causing five-hour disturbances. *She* thought that strange, since the facts suggested that an engagement reception of a Hindu engaged to a Christian was disturbed by thirty white youths who 'hurled petrol bombs through the downstairs windows forcing 80-odd guests from the Indian engagement party upstairs to protect themselves . . . of the 200 odd reported rioters, only 3 were arrested for violent disorder' (Gautama, 2001). *She* wondered how the petrol bombs just appeared and why a happy occasion should be turned into violent disorder while the police and others debate whether it had a racial motivation or not. 'Race' colours the judgement, like it or not. Shouldn't the violent disorder be appropriately dealt with, *She* asks?

She recalls in the last decade of the last century that although no violent disorders in social work took place, a campaign against anti-racism did. An attack on progress, nonetheless. A national strategy led by the UK body in social work, the Central Council for Education and Training in

Social Work (CCETSW) resulted in tangible progress in anti-racist social work arising from their policy commitment to implement the Race Relations Act 1976 as an education and a validating body.

Part I

'Time' has a way of creating coincidences: it was Sunday again. August 1st 1993. Just over a month to go before CCETSW disseminated the conclusion of its major Curriculum Development (CD) Project which resulted in seven training publications and produced twenty-eight writers, some black, some white, and none of whom had produced a training publication before. No time to be distracted or diverted *She* thought – one publication yet to be printed and a 120-person conference to be organised and managed. But there it was – the front page of *The Observer*: 'PC-anti-racist zealots drive away recruits', with more coverage inside by a respected journalist, M. Phillips. Anecdotal evidence from a handful of anonymous sources was presented as evidence of 'fear and intimidation' of lecturers in social work, who are being 'driven away' from their work and are 'in tears'. Other papers ran similar stories in the following days as did *The Independent* on 4 August with, 'Why paint so black a picture'? by B. Appleyard. His focus was on CCETSW's Paper 30 with its requirements for education and training in social work and on CCETSW's policy of anti-racism. The full page had a longer statement before the title: 'A social work directive elevates racism to a national epidemic. It is a national disgrace'.

She asked, is it so wrong to prepare social workers to better understand and to work competently with people from diverse communities? Racism exists – as does poverty – so is it so wrong to fight racism which affects people's lives in employment, in services and in training? Or was the purpose of the articles to assert that racism does not exist, so why all the fuss? *She* recalled that CCETSW's establishment of its anti-racism policy and of its requirements for trainers was no easy task, neither in relation to its introduction nor in its implementation. And yet the source of its reference was the Race Relations Act 1976. The changes made by CCETSW had their origins in grassroots support – a development that should have been seen as positive given that in the 1990s, and today in the new century, the emphasis is placed on user voice, and on consumer choice.

CCETSW was the first professional body to state as part of its requirements for courses to be approved that *all* social workers trained in the UK must be competent to work in a multiracial society. It followed from this competence requirement that social workers needed to be taught to understand racism and culture and develop appropriate skills. How else, *She* asks, can social workers form professional judgements in order to execute their role ? How can they case assess and manage users from different backgrounds other than their own? The irony *She* remembers in this period was that while CCETSW was attacked, as evidenced in the media campaign of 1993, at the same time the organisation was being asked by a range of bodies including the then Government, to give advice and access to use its materials. The health service, the police, the prison service and indeed the political parties were beginning to address the issues faced by black and minority ethnic people, as citizens, as employees, as students and as users.

The media campaign against CCETSW's policy and requirements in anti-racism was cloaked in the very same emotional language ('obsession', 'lethal kind of looniness') that, ironically, anti-racists are often accused of using.

None of the writers speaking out against CCETSW's stance ever disclosed their own position on racism, or offered any alternative strategy for the fight against racism. None suggested any ways in which services to black and minority ethnic communities could be designed and delivered. Their vague diatribes could not even be said to constitute sound journalism. For example, Phillips presents her argument as follows:

> in our University social work departments . . . the urge to stop oppression has itself become oppressive. Indeed, it would hardly be an exaggeration to describe what is going on as totalitarian . . . University tutors are abandoning social work teaching because they say they are being forced to teach 'political correctness' attitudes on race and gender in a climate of intimidation and fear.
>
> (*The Observer*, 1 August 1993)

Hughes (personal communication to the author, 1993) in responding to this article asked the paper's editor several questions:

> Who? How many lecturers are relinquishing their posts? At which Universities is this happening? Which social work professors are engaged in 'running battles' with CCETSW? In which particular Local Authorities' social services departments is the 'anti-racist preoccupation . . . depriving vulnerable clients of adequate standards of care'? What precisely does that mean? Just where are the institutions, in care, housing and education in which there is no evidence of under-representation of black and ethnic minority people in employment, or barriers to their access to services? These aren't difficult or unreasonable questions. They are the questions that any editor would ask of a journalist who tried to slip past the subs desk an article headlined, 'Anti-racist zealots "drive away recruits"'.

As in any area and particularly one concerning social conditions of human beings, mistakes do occur. The area of race relations is no different.

Indeed one may suggest that the pace and place of progress may be problematic because of lack of existing exemplars. In spite of this, as CCETSW showed, tangible progress rather than satisfaction with rhetoric can be accomplished. As some argued, perhaps this was the main reason for the media campaign. For others its purpose was to curtail the Council's independence and wanting to expose the then Health Minister Virginia Bottomley as 'soft' given her credentials in equality. Her inability to control CCETSW would diminish her status.[1] *She* however believed that the attack should be examined in a wider context: 'race' still strikes a chord with the masses (see for example, the *Daily Express* coverage of St George's Day and attack on the Commission for Racial Equality, 23 April 2001) and CCETSW's bold step in 'race' was therefore a weak link to the overall attack on social work education: education and social work were the two ideological frontiers and CCETSW stood alone, partly because other organisations had been previously attacked or closed down.

Patel acknowledges that:

> some serious mistakes have been made in the implementation of anti-racism programmes and these should be highlighted and changed. However, the many articles during the anti-CCETSW campaign of August/ September 1993 go beyond this. They have a number of themes in common: (1) there is an explicit denial that racism, and particularly institutionalised racism, exists (despite overwhelming evidence to the contrary; (2) amazingly, it is claimed that because antiracism declarations have been made (and surely these law-abiding Professors and journalists would want The Race Relations Act to be honoured – of which antiracism policies are but one product) the power balance has shifted so completely that the 'antiracism zealots' (presumably many of them black) are able to 'do things' to white tutors, practitioners and students;[2] and, finally, (3) 'the declarations are fine, but why do you want to implement them?' is a view which can be read between the lines of these articles. All the articles talk about how the requirements are '. . . inimical to open-minded inquiry and free speech.' How a 'climate of fear' is generated.
>
> (Patel, 1995: 40)

She thinks what is missed out in the flagrant attacks is:

1 consideration of the racism of the 1990s and its effects on services, communities and their ability to exercise their human rights; and
2 any appreciation that Paper 30, CCETSW's key document on requirements, which was the subject of their concern, could not be expected to be perfect, given the imperfections of the world it was written in.

Nevertheless the apparent impact of CCETSW's pronouncements examining the news coverage was that articles appeared to be fed with any line of opposition. Herein lies the depth of the problem. A question that could be legitimately asked is 'Who is being unethical?'. Some of the same journalists, a few years before these attacks on CCETSW had a record of speaking up for issues on 'race'. 'Remember race discussion? We used to worry about it once upon a time . . . We appear to have lost our sense of shame' (Phillips, 1988).

It was clear from this campaign against anti-racism that the 'creation of guilt charge' offered light to those who did not believe there was a need for service development and practice change to respond to Britain's diverse communities. Patel (1995) continues, 'Sivanandan (1988; 1993) is rightly critical of the Left who "accepted the spurious equation of individual growth with individualism and confuse personal moralism with socialist morality"' (1993: 18). Patel says, 'In the process their "right-on" thinking led them to coin "Politically Correct" language and behaviour, only to be hijacked by the Right and used as a vehicle for reactionary politics. Now those who stood for progress, for justice against racism and sexism, were openly charged with a "PC" label: a new form of McCarthyism had arrived, and the Right had found "an enemy within"'. Antiracism is regarded by the Right as a fanatical deviation' (1995: 41), but as Moore says: 'Western civilisation is not so fragile that it will crumble under the weight of a few black writers in the reading list, the odd exhibition by a female artist, a gay movie star – is it? Those who pit themselves against PC act as if they themselves had no agenda, as if they were entirely neutral forces simply protecting "our culture" from extremists. But ask yourself, as Mark Twain once did, "Who are you neutral against?"' (Moore, 1995: 5).

Part 2

Six years on in 1999, the hyperbole and rhetoric continued (as it does today in a new century) in the backlash against the Macpherson Report (1999) into the murder of a black teenager, Stephen Lawrence. *The Economist* described the report as representing a 'defining moment in race relations . . . by exposing the cancer of racism . . . it has stripped away any complacency that all is well' (27 February 1999). Yet papers like the *Daily Telegraph* have missed no opportunity to lambaste the Macpherson Report as described by Toynbee (1999). She quotes its editor, Charles Moore:

> You can be British without speaking English or being Christian or being white, but nevertheless Britain is basically English-speaking and Christian and white, and if one starts to think that it might become Urdu speaking and Muslim and brown, one gets frightened and angry. . . . Such feelings are not only natural, surely – they are right.
> (Toynbee, in *The Guardian*, 3 March 1999: 20)

Toynbee concludes:

> will anything change after Stephen Lawrence? Jack Straw and Tony
> Blair mean it to, but they are rolling stones uphill. The overwhelming
> press doesn't want change and all the institutional racists, witting and
> unwitting, will draw complacent comfort every day from reading their
> pages. No one's suggesting censoring them, but the Macpherson
> Report is becoming a rallying cry for Moore's vile vision of identity,
> nation and race. Let him call us politically correct: I call him a racist.
> (Ibid.)

And yet *She* thinks there is hope of action for progress. At the time of
CCETSW's closure, the 2001 census on 29 April is being carried out. It is
likely to show considerable variation in people of mixed parentage, of
people born in Britain and the fact that the UK's minorities are creating
and contributing to Britain as they have always done. The likes of people
Toynbee describes will have to contend with the economics of a demography
that is likely to be very mixed indeed. How black and minority ethnic people
themselves respond will also impact as will the larger social and economic
changes in our society along with policies on regeneration, social inclusion
and development.

CCETSW did make considerable progress in spite of a poor climate for
change. The campaign against anti-racism also had specific impact on individuals leading the initiative within and without. As an organisation, those
in charge worked hard to maintain the progress in spite of the campaign
against anti-racism. There are lessons to be learned both from this intense
experience of implementing anti-racism requirements, and from the situation
of an attack on CCETSW's progress in a context where that progress had
been commended by the then Government.

Some of the lessons concern how the social care sector itself responds, or
not. Several prominent academics in social work and beyond (Dominelli,
Jones, Triseliotis and others) did write in the national press on the usefulness
of the anti-racism requirements in their role as educators – and perhaps many
others did whose contribution did not get published. But a question remains
– *She* remembers the perception that many were willing to 'counsel' rather
than be proactively involved to address the imbalance in the campaign
against anti-racism. For some, the campaign justified their resistance and
gave it a degree of plausibility in terms of why they should 'go slow' on
CCETSW's anti-racism requirements. As the coverage described earlier in
2001 suggests, the same issues recur on 'race'. Social care educators and
students of the care professions are at the forefront of working to develop
and improve practices to help those who are disadvantaged and discriminated against – in order to make a difference to their lives. Can we today
be confident that if a similar campaign against anti-racism ensued those in

charge of it would keep their nerve and defend the rights of people whom it serves?

The new bodies in social care, TOPSS, City and Guilds, SCIE, GSSC and indeed social care employers such as ADSS/ADSW and LGA[3] need to ask of themselves how they are meeting (will meet) the real issues faced by black and minority ethnic people in mental health, children, older people's services, for example. The issues of 'race' and anti-racism in the implementation of CCETSW's requirements were not divorced from these realities: this is what the issue of 'race' is all about (Lord Dholakia, interviewed in Channel 4 News, 23 April 2001).

She reminds us how history suggests the need to recognise progress and to build upon it, employing appropriate strategies to reflect the changing circumstances and challenges. For example one of the major achievements was in relation to the pioneering of education materials that moved beyond the rhetorical level and that gave examples of addressing racism in practice. In 1998 when CCETSW endorsed the policy on anti-racism and reflected this in its requirements, there was no training publication in the social care sector in working in different areas of care with black and minority ethnic clients. At the end of the three-phase Curriculum Development (CD) Project in 1993, seven publications were produced involving 400 people. Twenty-eight members were organised into six subject areas: working with children and families; elders; mental health; learning disability; criminal justice; and practice teaching, with these members becoming the authors of the publications. They were women and men, practitioners and academics and, as noted earlier, both black and white. The first publication was *Setting the Context for Change* (1990). This was an edited book aiming to provide understanding of the general issues in 'race' and racism and with an applied section on social work education and practice.

At the end of the CD Project's life Patel, who created and managed it with support from a steering group, undertook a small-scale research study into the project's design and its impact on members. Members were asked if the project principles, including multiracial and collective working, mattered to them in three respects:

- organising their group;
- its operation; and
- the product.

In all three cases the sixteen respondents gave a firm 'yes', a unanimous agreement.

The building of the CD Project infrastructure took place prior to Phase 1: the ship,[4] (speaking as a non-sailor), was launched in October 1988 with Phase 1; made a maiden voyage in Phase 2 and fully filled with people in

Phase 3. Its course was charted and roles and responsibilities agreed upon, but it was hard to gauge how it would arrive at its ultimate destination, negotiate rough seas, and long becalmed periods because of poor wind, or respond to some team members jumping overboard. After all, this was no ordinary sea it sailed and one that had seldom been crossed successfully. Occasionally, the sails needed to be reset and many types of people set the ship back on course. Sometimes letters were sent when rumours stirred among the sailing teams that the steering team was going to run away with their booty to Brazil! Every year, beginning with 1991, each sailing crew got an award and then, in 1993, the ship with its six-fold crew and the steering team docked, carrying seven treasure chests amid the cheering crowds at St Anne's-on-Sea in September 1993.

Epilogue

The ship, the CD Project, put into port having achieved what it had set out to do, with the method and principles upheld. One of the co-authors and a convenor of a core group wrote about his experience and analysis of the CD Project, which is worth quoting in this context:

> Looking back, the CD Project represented some kind of 'new social movement' in which, in Audre Lorde's terms, differences were acknowledged and even celebrated and used as a force for change. We were united by recognition of the need for anti-racist change at all levels, including, crucially, the curriculum, and we developed some kind of collective action, which transcended hierarchies of white/black, teacher/student, and academic/practitioner. The CD texts are both a process and a product containing, for all their faults, innovative curriculum material. For all of the missed deadlines, disagreements, and recriminations, they were enjoyable to produce and the web of inter-relationships which lay behind them were of immense importance in developing a network of anti-racists able and willing to be called upon, reciprocally, as external examiners, witnesses in industrial tribunals, and, even, simply as someone to talk to at times when you thought you were going mad. In contrast to the Warwick experience, here was a kind of social praxis of which, I like to think, Freire would be proud.
>
> (Stubbs, 1995, unpublished ms)

Interestingly the economics of demography and business are pointing to the necessity of valuing multiracial working. Thus *The Economist* reported:

> according to an article in the current issue of the *Academy of Management Journal* . . . Press disclosures that firms discriminate against

women or minorities soon result in a fall in the share price . . . Firms with a good track record of producing non-white managers and managing people from different backgrounds will enjoy a growing advantage in recruiting and motivating workers. They may also be more attuned to an increasingly diverse population of customers. Equally, firms, which continue to favour white men, will find themselves fishing in a shrinking pool of potential employees. Most intriguingly, ethnic diversity may help American firms outperform their rivals abroad.

The CD Project shattered some myths: that black and white cannot work successfully together; that collective working is neither possible nor needed; and that academics and practitioners cannot work together. In practice much anti-racist work is not taken up or published. The CD Project made it central and achieved not one, but seven publications, all regarded as important source material in education and training of social workers. The rising sales of these publications demonstrated just how popular they were. The CD Project was an original idea that was fragile, not in content or form, but in the very process of being set up in an organisation within which, with its many aims and constraints (and usual decision-making processes), a good idea could have been easily lost. But it overcame that fragility and moved from aims, to action, to publication and to dissemination, having retained the integrity of the original idea throughout its five-year life.

The challenge, and indeed the opportunity for the present and emerging generation of social work students, trainers and workers, is one of how to safeguard what has been hard won and learned in an area that expresses the realities of disadvantage, discrimination and diversity so clearly among its 'client base'. Amid this, it has to manage the resistance and the kind of attacks that have been described in this chapter in order to protect – and hold out the possibility of improving – the futures of all those working in the field. Clarity of aims, understanding of racism and its impact on services and social work practice for the various communities, a non-doctrinaire approach in 'race' and social work (elsewhere *She* remembers critique of those who personalise racism and equate it to guilt and the rising focus on identity rather than day-to-day issues of care, safety, jobs, services) with qualities of perseverance, determination and good strategic planning and implementation are the hallmarks of progress in bringing about racial and social justice (Patel 1995). There is also the critique on the preference for a 'checklist' approach in social care, which, while understandable particularly given the pressures on the staff, produces 'stagnant thinking'. The approach suggested is thus:

> good practice that is sensitive to the needs of minority clients means adopting an open-ended approach. Being receptive to situations

rather than putting situations in a pre-designed framework is the good that we should strive for.

(Patel, 2001: 168)

The campaign against anti-racism today continues to be characterised by the same features that have been described in relation to the attack on CCETSW. The focus is on making 'race' a constant issue when in reality as Hughes (1993) said in his letter on the Phillips article, 'the reality is that there is probably no story here worth publishing in a national newspaper. "Professor Pinker and a handful of academics disagree with accrediting body", is a real "Man wonders about biting dog", sort of story'.

The work and benefits brought about to make sure that social care meets the needs of Britain's diverse population deserves serious consideration, examining approaches and ideas that best meet them rather than whether there is an issue of 'race' racism to be addressed or not. Racism is as real as poverty. We choose to change or not. That is the power we have as professionals, as educators and as decision makers.

Notes

1 The genesis of the media campaign is in 1992. G. Hartup writing in *Freedom Today* (1992), a magazine published by the Freedom Association said, 'capture of social work by a coalition of Marxists, feminists and anti-racists had put the fruits of their ten year struggle at risk. . . . Utilising our research, *Sunday Times* columnist Barbara Amiel wrote a brilliant polemic attacking Virginia Bottomley (11 October 1992). Ms Amiel repeated that attack at greater length in *The Spectator* (19 October 1992) basing it on a speech at a fringe meeting of the Centre for Policy Studies at the Conservative Conference (8 October 1992)'.
2 This situation must have completely passed me by. From experience we know that anti-racism issues can be magnified by an individual's view of the world. Obviously, this generates a lot of feeling and emotional response – but which area of the human condition does not? What is at stake is that social work professionals and students are in the thick of dealing with humans – and anti-racist knowledge is one of the key skills in being a competent social worker.
3 TOPSS = Training Organisations in Personal Social Services; SCIE = Social Care Institute of Excellence; GSSC = General Social Services Council; ADSS = Association of Directors of Social Services; ADSW = Association of Directors of Social Work (Scotland); LGA = Local Government Association; CCETSW = Central Council for Education and Training in Social Work.
4 Thanks to Dr Martin Willis at Birmingham University, for suggesting this metaphor.

References

Appleyard, B. (1993) 'Why paint so black a picture?' *The Independent*, 4 August.
Gautama, P. (2001) 'Attacks in Bradford', *Gujarat Samachar*, 21 April.
Macpherson, W. (1999) *The Stephen Lawrence Enquiry*, London: Stationery Office.

Patel, N. (1995) 'In search of the holy grail', in Hugman, R. and Smith, D. (eds) *Ethical Issues in Social Work*, London: Routledge.

Patel, N. (2001) 'Minority ethnic elderly, ageing with care', in Dominelli, L., Lorenz, W. and Soydan, H. (eds) *Beyond Racial Divides – Ethnicities in Social Work Practice*, Aldershot: Ashgate.

Phillips, M. (1988) 'How Britain still plays the white man', *The Guardian*, 24 June.

Phillips, M. (1993) 'PC-antiracist zealots drive away recruits', *The Observer*, 1 August.

Chapter 3

Developing anti-discriminatory practice

Neil Thompson

Introduction

Anti-discriminatory practice has established itself as a mainstay of social work education over the past fifteen years or so, and is increasingly featuring in the professional education of health care workers and others within the human services. It has to be recognised that, although considerable progress has been made, the process has not been an easy or trouble-free one, and continues to be problematic in some ways. In this chapter, I therefore seek to build on the strengths and to guard against the problems. In order to do this I have divided the chapter into three main sections. In the first, I ask the question: what is anti-discriminatory practice? Given that this is something of a contested area of enquiry, I begin with some scene setting and briefly outline my own views of what anti-discriminatory practice is and why it is important. In the second section, I explore the question of how we make it a reality, taking account of the complex relationships across the personal and broader cultural and structural dimensions of discrimination (Thompson, 2001). Finally, in the third section, I identify some of the main pitfalls to avoid. This involves exploring a range of issues relating to how our attempts to promote anti-discriminatory practice can be flawed and at times counterproductive.

What is anti-discriminatory practice?

The basis of anti-discriminatory practice can be understood in terms of a sequence, with each of the following four terms linked to the next one in the 'chain': from diversity to difference through to discrimination and oppression. I shall explain each in turn.

Diversity

I use this term in its quite literal sense to refer to the fact that society is characterised by immense variation. Although there are very many similarities and commonalities that can be identified, it remains the case that there are huge differences to be found not only across social groups but also within them. Society reflects this diversity in so far as social groups tend continually to form and reform around aspects of identity they have in common such as: religion or creed; 'community' or identification with a locality; occupation or vocation; and a wide array of leisure and recreational lifestyles. The range of these identities is extensive, and innumerable subtle distinctions can be drawn both between and within the social groups that are formed. Diversity is to be found as much among, say, 'travellers' – people who do not follow sedentary, settled living patterns, as among the 'domiciled' – people who do. It is distinctions such as these that provide a starting point for investigating this topic.

The contemporary emphasis on promoting, affirming or even celebrating diversity – the 'diversity approach', as it has come to be known – is, in part, a recognition of the changes in British culture that are associated with the development of what Rex (1996) has called 'moderate multiculturalism'. As Bonnett (2000) has shown, at other points in history such diversity was construed unequivocally as presenting, in its own right, a threat to political and social unity, to the feeling of togetherness or of national community. By contrast, the emphasis of the promoting diversity approach is that the existence of a diverse population is, in itself, seen as an asset, rather than a problem requiring a solution. Diversity is seen as the basis of a society enriched by the variety of differences across the population. Anti-discriminatory practice therefore involves recognising and promoting the value of diversity.

Difference

Diversity is based on difference – that is, it is the range of differences in society that add up to form the backcloth of diversity. Such differences can be conceptualised in two important ways in relation to diversity. First, difference can be seen in terms of the classic social divisions of class, gender, race, ethnicity, disability, sexual orientation and so on, as well as other less well-documented social categories and boundaries. Second, it can be understood in terms of social reality being in a constant state of flux, such perpetual change reflecting the ways in which people continually adapt to circumstances. That is, a recognition of difference as an important issue involves a move away from 'essentialism' – the view of individuals as fixed and immutable identities. I shall return to this point below.

The notion of difference as an important issue is closely associated with poststructuralist and postmodernist thought in which social differences are recognised as fundamental elements of the social order and the nature of social reality (Stewart, 2001).

Discrimination

The point that should be emphasised here is that, wherever there is difference, there is the potential for discrimination. In its literal sense, the word 'discriminate' means to delineate or identify a difference. That is, to discriminate, in its general sense, is an essential part of social interaction, and indeed of making sense of our lives. While it may seem a simple and obvious point to grasp, it should be made clear that it is therefore a particular type of discrimination that is being specified when we look at anti-discriminatory practice – a quite specific and negative type of unfair, oppressive discrimination. What is in question here, then, are those forms of discrimination that lead to particular individuals and/or groups being discriminated against and thus suffering a disadvantage – or, to use the legal term, a detriment. This is where the fourth term, that of oppression, comes in, as it is through being disadvantaged and discriminated against that people experience oppression.

Oppression

What is at issue here is the range of situations where discrimination takes place in unfair, inappropriate, and destructive ways which have oppressive consequences for the people who are discriminated against. This involves recognising that discrimination is not simply unfair, in a narrow, ethical sense, but also a major source of disadvantage, pain, suffering and degradation – in short, oppression.

It is unfortunately the case that those people who see anti-discriminatory practice as a threat to their own position of power and privilege will often attempt to counter it by deploying the 'positive' aspects of the term discrimination. Thus it will be argued that people are of course different, and are going to be discriminated between and against – that is reality, it is part of human nature. However, this is to oversimplify the relationship between discrimination and oppression.

As Mishra (1995) points out, although, in many senses, the arguments against discrimination on the basis of gender, disability and ethnicity, have been accepted by UK and other European governments, the arguments for equality have not. The acceptance of inequality means that it is considered fair to discriminate against, for example, those who do not fit in with the economic imperative of a flexible labour market because they are unable, or unwilling to be flexible in finding and keeping work – indeed, such discrimination is endorsed. This can lead to a 'naturalising' of social inequality, in which such discrimination is presented as natural and indeed necessary for social and economic stability. It is part of the conservative and liberal traditions of social thought for it to be regarded as legitimate for social groups to engage in discriminatory actions within circumscribed areas, such as work, health and personal relationships, within certain limits, and by legal means (Thompson and Thompson, 1993). The process and act of negative discrimination are masked, and even justified, by the ideology of competitive individualism which supports this oppression and is presented as a positive facet of society.

It is important to note that some commentators, such as Phillipson (1992), make a distinction between anti-discriminatory and anti-oppressive practice, reserving the former for relatively narrow, legalistic approaches to these issues. In terms of the approach that I am outlining in this chapter, it should be recognised that I regard the two terms as referring to the same thing. Whether attempts are made to stop the discrimination that leads to the oppression, or to deal with the resulting oppression, the primary objective in practice remains broadly the same. One of my concerns is that it is very easy for people who are part of the same anti-oppressive movement to end up fighting each other over terminology. We do, of course have to be clear about what we mean, and so care needs to be taken to present our ideas with as much clarity as possible.

In sum, then, my answer to the question of 'what is anti-discriminatory practice?' is that it is any form of practice that tries to prevent the recognition of difference being used as the basis of unfair discrimination, leading to oppressive consequences for people. The starting point is the recognition of diversity as an asset, a positive advantage rather than a problem, and difference, equally, as something that can bestow benefits. From this point, the legitimate need to discriminate between people can be separated from processes of unfair, unjust or destructive comparison, so that we do not reach the position of oppression.

Unless we take seriously the dangers of unfair discrimination being allowed to lead to oppression, we run the risk of failing in our duty of care, with the possible outcome that our interventions do more harm than good. It is therefore important to have at least a basic grasp of the complexities of making anti-discriminatory practice a reality, and so it is to this that we now turn.

How do we make anti-discriminatory practice a reality?

To address this question, I shall draw on what I refer to as 'PCS analysis' (Thompson, 2001). Put succinctly, PCS analysis is a framework which breaks down the complex issues of discrimination into three separate but inter-related levels: Personal, Cultural and Structural. The basis of PCS analysis is that any approaches to the questions of discrimination and oppression which do not take account of all three of these levels, and their inter-relationships, is in danger of oversimplifying a very complex set of issues. I shall explain, in turn, what is meant by each of the three terms, personal, cultural and structural.

Personal

A key objective of developing a multidimensional approach is to address the problem that so often occurs where people see only the personal aspects of discrimination: a person is seen as being a 'racist', or a 'chauvinist', for example – as if it were simply a matter of personal qualities. Discrimination is very often represented simply as the manifestation of a set of personal prejudices, attitudes of bigotry that are seen as part of the individual's psychological make-up. Of course, for some people, discriminatory views are indeed a significant part of their personal identity – members of extremist racialist organisations, for example. But the limitation of such an approach to the issue of discrimination is that it often leads other people to rely on statements such as: 'I'm not prejudiced, so this is not an issue for me', as if there is nothing more to consider than personal prejudice or personal views on the subject.

The key point is that the cultural and structural levels always operate in tandem with the personal level. Even if racism is not a significant part of a particular individual's persona or attitudes on a personal level, it will nonetheless remain an issue to be addressed at the cultural and structural levels with which we all engage, on a continuous basis, whether or not we are aware of it. We are all part of the networks of shared meanings and discourses that form the cultural level and the networks of power and social standing that form the structural level. Personal prejudice is, therefore, part of the complex web of discrimination, but we should be wary of overestimating its importance and thus underestimating the significance of cultural and structural factors

Cultural

In describing the cultural level, I use culture in an anthropological sense to apply to the entire set of belief systems of a society. That is, I am not confining my idea of culture to that of specific sets of moral beliefs and values. PCS analysis does not relate only to culture in the sense of religious, national or ethnic background. I use the term, rather, to refer to a set of shared meanings, where people use language and imagery in a particular way to produce a 'discourse' – a set of ideas and meanings that come as a package. Embedded within these sets of ideas and meanings are images of what certain groups in society are like, and how they are expected to behave. These images are often inaccurate and carry discriminatory connotations about those that they represent.

Stereotypes are an important feature of the cultural level. Righton (1990) makes a useful distinction between 'typifications' and 'stereotypes' in respect of the images of people that are presented within discourse. A typification is a set of expectations that we have about a person, a group or a thing. As long as these expectations are provisional, and provide us with a guide which we change and update with experience, then our typifications are a helpful means of breaking down the complexity of social reality. But, when we are dealing with a stereotype, on the other hand, problems of discrimination come to the fore. A stereotype is a fixed and unchanging set of expectations we hold on to because our sense of personal security may be threatened if they are thrown into question. As Righton (1990) explains:

> The trouble comes when we become so emotionally attached to a par-
> ticular typification that we experience any questioning of it as a threat
> to our self-esteem or sense of security, or as a challenge to the power
> we hold. We will then tend to cling desperately to that typification
> come what may, however strong the contradictory evidence. When
> this happens, the typification – now fixed and rigid – has become
> what we call a stereotype.
>
> (Cited in Thompson, 2001: 27)

One relevant example of a stereotype is that of the 'immigrant community' which figured strongly in the political and cultural discourse of the 1950s and 1960s in Britain (Abbott, 1971). The counterposing of the 'immigrant' to the 'host' community in language played a key role in defining the status of the respective parties involved. The white majority community was the host, and the black and Asian immigrant, minority communities were the guests. An implication of this terminology was that the immigrant did not have a right to belong in the host society and was, rather, a temporary visitor who should not abuse the hospitality offered. The white community was portrayed as 'settled' and characterised by togetherness and belonging. Immigrants, on the other hand, were presented as having problems of adapt-ing to this settled community on account of their different backgrounds and expectations. Divisions within the host community were thus obscured within this discourse.

The 'host community' was, throughout this period, itself highly stratified and characterised by very significant inequalities of wealth, power and status between social classes. As Crompton (1993: 193) comments, all of the various 'heuristic maps' of sociological analysis have identified a 'persist-ing concentration of economic, organisational and political power within an "upper class" which comprises only a small minority of the population'. This 'majority' problem of difference is generally and conveniently forgotten in the discourse of ethnic difference at the cultural level, a tendency which is still apparent even in the more socially 'inclusive' policy which holds at the time of writing (Burden and Hamm, 2000).

Language use is also an important aspect of the cultural level. For example, language is important in reinforcing attitudes to, and beliefs about, older people. Fennell *et al.* (1988: 7) comment that they try, as teachers and writers, to avoid using terms such as 'the elderly', 'geriatrics, the elderly mentally infirm', 'the old' or 'the confused'. This is not in an attempt to deny that there are physical and mental changes in old age, but rather 'to try, linguistically, to remind ourselves constantly of human variety in the groups we are categorising and to underline the "people status" (people like us in other words) of elderly people as opposed to the "thing status" (objects inferior to us) of "the elderly"'. Thus they regard 'older people' and 'people in old age' as preferable terms to 'the elderly'.

This kind of debate is often seen as obsessively 'PC' – that is to say, it is seen to be over concerned with the objective of political correctness. But, as I will discuss further below, the attribution of negative labels to different social groups can have a serious impact on the self-image of those concerned, especially where the term is used regularly in addressing the group and acts to reinforce the perception of helplessness, uselessness and dependency of its members. Just as significant are the messages which the use of negative labels gives to others, in terms of a linguistic licence to regard the groups concerned as inferior. It is therefore clear that it is not politically (or morally) correct to those to whom the labels are attached. The journal *Disability and Society* comments, in this respect that:

> although, 'disabled people and their organisations have . . . drawn attention to the problem of offensive language, . . . there remains less general awareness of the ways in which words are used to stigmatise and discriminate against people with impairments.
>
> (Executive Editors, 1993: 109–10)

For this reason, the phrase 'disabled people', the journal suggests, is increasingly used by those who are referred to in order 'to convey a positive identity'.

The use of terminology is very important in constructing social identities as Foucault (1977, 1979) has shown. Language is not an inert container of words that we pick up and use as the occasion demands, but something that is active and dynamic within the social world.

Unquestioned assumptions are a further aspect of the cultural level. For example, Hockey and James (1993: 13) refer to the problem of 'infantilisation', the tendency to treat older people as if they were children. They argue that 'the cultural pervasiveness and embeddedness of metaphors of childhood within the discourses surrounding ageing and dependency' allow views about what are appropriate ways of looking after children to be 'unquestioningly and "naturally" transferred to other dependent groups'.

It is therefore important in health and social services to counter these processes, and one means of doing so is what Sartre (1963) referred to as the 'progressive–regressive method'. Older people as recipients of services have a repertoire of past roles, problems and choices of direction which give a means of orientation. These factors also constitute a part of the self with which there can be interaction in order for future roles to be developed. What one has been can be reconstructed to guide what one will be (Thompson, 1998b). Throughout our existence we each have a past that we can look back on (the regressive element) and a future that we can anticipate (the progressive element). We should therefore avoid the ageist assumption that older people have a past but no future. What each of us faces in the future is the rest of our life and it is precisely that, the rest of our life, however long or short that may be for the individual concerned. Consequently, in relation to older people, it can clearly be seen that anti-discriminatory practice connects the way we use language, as an aspect of the cultural level, to the ways we recognise and address the social 'markers' of age, and to the ways that we accord significance to the inner conflicts and concerns of those who are the clients of services.

Structural

Mention of these social 'markers' of ageing, such as loss of power and influence, takes us to the structural level. Of course, it is no coincidence that there are so many powerful assumptions, sets of meanings and images operating at the cultural level to reinforce power relations in society. Discrimination operates at that level in terms of institutionalised power relationships. Taking gender and sexism, as one important example, it is recognised that positions of power in organisations are predominantly held by men (Abbott and Wallace, 1997). Equally, in respect of racism, the cultural cues for racial discrimination to take place are associated with the fact that powerful positions in society are overwhelmingly held by white people (Small, 1994).

Power, at a structural level, can be seen to follow the 'fault lines' of society that is, to reflect the social divisions of class, race, ethnicity, gender, age, disability and so on. Power is not equally distributed across the structure of society, and indeed the structured nature of society gives some groups more power at the expense of others (for example, in relation to class and poverty – Jones and Novak, 1999).

The cultural factors both reflect and reinforce the structural basis of society – the power relations that underpin it. Recognising discrimination is therefore not simply a matter of identifying a specific piece of behaviour or action, it is more a matter of appreciating the continuous interplay of all three levels. PCS analysis is a dynamic model of this interaction, and that is one of the reasons why it is so complex, and why one of the dangers is that of oversimplification, as I shall discuss below.

Within PCS analysis, ideology can be seen as the glue that binds the levels together: it is transmitted from the cultural level to the personal level, from where it is reflected back again, and it is transmitted to the structural level to underpin social divisions and the distribution of power in society. In this process, the effect of ideology is to allow the structural divisions to appear 'normal' and for people thus routinely to accept them without great question. For example, at the structural level, the 'feminisation of poverty' (Millar, 1989), a process characterised by the salience of women's employment profile in poorly paid, insecure, part-time work, is considered to be a consequence of females, especially in their roles as mothers, *naturally* having less interest in the world of work outside the home.

Before leaving the subject of PCS analysis, a cautionary note about the use of this framework is called for. In the period since I first wrote about PCS analysis in the early 1990s, and in the course of my work as an external examiner for Diploma in Social Work programmes, I have seen very many essays that cite the concept in their argument but do not actually make any use of it – they simply name it, rather than use it as an analytical frame-work. Unfortunately, it would seem that many of its student admirers do not actually recognise the significance of what it means and how it can be used as a basis for promoting anti-discriminatory practice. Thus tutors often write in the margin of these essays, at the points where PCS analysis is mentioned: 'Why? Explain this', 'How is it useful?' and so on. I am therefore very concerned that this might, if used in this way, become a form of 'mantra', a magic phrase to incant when, of course, it is not intended as any such thing. It is a conceptual tool developed as a foundation for understanding the complexities involved.

So, in response to the second of the questions I set myself at the beginning of this chapter, 'how do we make it a reality?', my argument is that we do so by addressing all three levels wherever possible. A strategy that simply tries to identify certain individuals who have discriminatory attitudes that need to be addressed can leave structures, assumptions and powerful meanings in place and will be far from adequate. This is not to say that there should be no attention to individuals whose views are unacceptable, but it is to say that it is not enough on its own to tackle personal issues – it is also necessary to look at the cultural and structural contexts in which they are embedded.

What are the pitfalls to avoid?

In addressing this question, I am concerned with looking at how strategies can go wrong and some of the common difficulties that present themselves.

This is a major topic and so I shall limit myself to examining seven possible pitfalls, namely: essentialism; reductionism; dogmatism; determinism; defensiveness; 'non-dialectical' approaches; and drift.

Essentialism

The basis of essentialism is the belief that people are best understood as fixed entities, with our personality based on unchanging 'essences' which make us what we are. For example, if a person is perceived as a racist, then this is regarded as an unchanging quality which forms part of that person's identity.

One of the clear problems with such an approach is that it oversimplifies the situation, and attributes discriminatory attitudes to certain people being seen as 'bad' individuals, rather than taking into account the broader issues of the cultural and structural dimensions discussed above. For example, some people may behave in a discriminatory way in certain circumstances but not in others. A male school teacher who, while at school, is very committed to trying to challenge sexist or racist (or any other form) of discriminatory stereotypes and works very hard to avoid reinforcing discrimination may, when outside school – for example, when socialising with friends – indulge in all sorts of racist and sexist jokes and banter. The idea that an individual either is or is not a discriminatory person is therefore far too simplistic. It is always necessary to look more broadly at the circumstances.

Reductionism

This is closely related to essentialism and describes the situation where a phenomenon that has many aspects to it is reduced to one aspect, thus representing part of an explanation as if it were the whole. There may be a particular event which is part of a complex picture, but in the account of what happens, the rest of that situation is not taken into account – it is only that one aspect that is seen as significant.

For example, the situation may occur where women within a team consider that the reason they do not appear to be listened to by management is to do with sexist discriminatory perceptions of them held by male managers. Such explanations, which may hold some truth in them, run the risk – if taken as sufficient in themselves – of ignoring key facets of organisational culture in which a number of key issues around gender and other dimensions of power are likely to feature strongly. This broader context of the setting for suggestions to managers will also be worthy of consideration if we are trying to understand the apparent rejection of women's views, in terms of how 'helpful' or otherwise the comments put forward are considered to be (Dearlove, 1973; Cochrane, 1993).

Dogmatism

This is represented by the idea that there is only one true answer in these matters, and that a person is either right or wrong. Indeed, positivist approaches in the social sciences support dogmatism to the extent that they operate on the premise that research will eventually uncover principles of how human interaction works, in all circumstances, and that, as a consequence, the 'right' thing to do in terms of managing that interaction will be discernible (Crook *et al.*, 1992). However, as I have suggested in discussing what social work can learn from other disciplines (Thompson and Bates, 1996), the concept of reflective practice indicates how the tendency to dogmatism can be addressed (see also Thompson, 2000a). Reflective practice encourages self-criticism and recognises that the professional repertoire of techniques will not always be adequate to the task in hand. Novel problems for the practitioner will require a re-thinking of standard approaches. Equally, anti-discriminatory practice involves very complex and highly political issues, to which there is often no 'textbook' answer. The fact that one person's way of addressing them may be different from another's does not mean that one is necessarily right and the other necessarily wrong. There are different approaches that may all have some degree of validity – there is, of course, no single definitive right answer.

Determinism

This refers to the belief that people are not responsible for their own actions, and that discriminatory attitudes are predetermined by factors such as social upbringing, and therefore cannot be helped. A deterministic attitude is also one where the individual regards the addressing of social problems and solutions as primarily a broader social responsibility rather than a personal matter. This is reflected in the view that inequality is inevitable. If society is based on inequality, then this is a fact that simply has to be accepted and lived with. If an individual does not occupy a position of privilege within the dominant power structures – that is, he or she is outside the corridors of power, as most of us are – then it is not possible for that person to do anything to change the circumstances. The individual is regarded as being powerless to change anything. Seeing powerlessness as inevitable then represents a denial of the relevance of the principles of citizenship, of civil, political, and social rights that have been developed as a basis of the 'welfare state' (Cochrane and Clarke, 1993). In terms of PCS analysis, it means that, as with essentialism, the personal is once again being separated from the cultural and structural levels.

Defensiveness

Again, it should be borne in mind that anti-discriminatory practice involves highly complex, highly political issues. It is understandable that some people may become very nervous and anxious when it comes to tackling these issues. I have noted above that there are many reasons for defensiveness, ranging from attachment to a typification, which has become a stereotype for the person concerned and which plays a role in his or her emotional security and self-regard, to antipathy towards what may be seen as 'political correctness'. In particular, white males, who generally hold the positions of power in health and welfare services, may be expected to be defensive for that reason. It is very important to go beyond defensiveness, because these are major issues in people's lives, and this barrier has to be overcome if progress is to be made in addressing patterns of oppression and discrimination.

'Non-dialectical' approaches

A dialectical approach is one that is characterised by three main elements (Thompson, 1998a):

- It is dynamic. This means that it recognises that a static, once-and-for-all analysis is inadequate – human existence is characterised by change and movement.
- It is interactive. The interaction of conflicting forces (the efforts of different interest groups, such as social classes, for example) is also a feature of human existence and the social context in which it takes place.
- It totalises. This means that it takes account of a wide range of factors and does not rely on one or two aspects alone (see the discussion of reductionism above).

A non-dialectical approach is therefore one which falls down in one or more of these respects. Perhaps the most common form of non-dialectical approach is where people try to develop simple solutions to complex problems – for example, by producing a list of 'taboo' words that should be avoided, rather than by developing a sensitivity to the complex role of language and its interaction with other aspects of the situation being dealt with.

Drift

I use this term in a particular sense to describe a barrier to good practice in general. At times practitioners and managers in health and social services can become so busy that they lose sight of what they are trying to achieve – they 'lose the plot' (Thompson, 1996). This can apply in two senses, the general and the specific. In general, it means that people can become so busy that they lose the focus of their workload, they no longer have a clear vision of what they are trying to achieve or how they are going to achieve it. It can also apply specifically when people lose sight of the objectives of anti-discriminatory practice, with the result that the means become the end. This problem of drift and lack of focus is aptly captured in the following comment from Brandon which echoes my comments earlier about the oversimplified use of PCS analysis:

> Anti-discrimination strategies become ends in themselves, just mantras for use in college student assignments, separated from any genuine struggle against racism or sexism. We lose sight of the overall struggle for liberation.
>
> (Brandon, 2000: 56)

Similarly, Collins (2001) gives some useful illustrations of this tendency within NHS Trusts. Human resources managers within Trusts often carry out detailed work to develop policies on bullying and racial harassment, but then may neglect the organisational environment of those policies. The policies and procedures once again become an end in themselves, and therefore do not necessarily contribute to a workplace characterised by the notion of 'dignity at work' (Thompson, 2000b). In such cases, a question that needs to be regularly asked and, more importantly, answered is this: 'is it safe for staff to complain of harassment in our current organisational environment and culture?'.

Conclusion

Here I return to the questions I set out at the beginning of the chapter. In answer to the first question 'what is anti-discriminatory practice?', I have argued that it is any form of action that tries to prevent the sequence from diversity to difference to discrimination and on to oppression. In answer to the second question, that of how we make anti-discriminatory practice a reality, I have indicated that it is by recognising that it is a complex set of issues that can be seen to operate at personal, cultural and structural levels, and that we must try to address all three of those levels wherever possible. In terms of how we avoid our attempts going wrong, I have argued that there is a need to look carefully at the pitfalls that are always lying in wait to divert us away from the objectives of anti-discriminatory practice, such as determinism, essentialism and defensiveness.

Developing anti-discriminatory practice is not a simple matter, nor is it something that can be done in a short period of time. What is required is a commitment to wrestling with the complexities, learning the difficult lessons and being prepared to take the necessary steps over an extended period of time. This is a major undertaking, but one that is necessary if we are serious about not allowing discrimination and oppression to undermine our efforts to support people through the problems and challenges they face.

References

Abbot, P. and Wallace, C. (1997) *An Introduction to Sociology: Feminist Perspectives*, London: Routledge.

Abbott, S. (ed.) (1971) *The Prevention of Racial Discrimination in Britain*, London: Oxford University Press.

Bonnett, A. (2000) *White Identities*, Harlow: Pearson.

Brandon, D. (2000) *The Tao of Survival: Spirituality in Social Care and Counselling*, Birmingham: Venture Press.

Burden, T. and Hamm, T. (2000) 'Responding to socially excluded groups', in Percy-Smith, J. (ed.) (2000) *Policy Responses to Social Exclusion: Towards Inclusion?*, Buckingham: Open University Press.

Cochrane, A. (1993) *Whatever Happened to Local Government?* Buckingham: Open University Press.

Cochrane, A. and Clarke, J. (1993) *Comparing Welfare States: Britain In International Context*, London: Sage.

Collins, M. (2001) 'Good practice, networks and the NHSE programme: the plan for action to tackle harassment and bullying in the NHS', paper delivered to a conference on anti-discriminatory practice and equal opportunities, University of Leeds, 10 January.

Crompton, R. (1993) *Class and Stratification: An Introduction to Current Debates*, Cambridge: Polity Press.

Crook, S., Pakulski, J. and Waters, M. (1992) *Postmodernization: Change in Advanced Society*, London: Sage.

Dearlove, J. (1973) *The Politics of Policy in Local Government: The Making and Maintenance of Public Policy in the Royal Borough of Kensington and Chelsea*, Falmer: University of Sussex.

Executive Editors (1993) 'Editorial', *Disability, Handicap and Society*, vol. 8, no. 2.

Fennell, G., Phillipson, C. and Evers, H. (1988) *The Sociology of Old Age*, Buckingham: Open University Press.

Foucault, M. (1977) *Discipline and Punish: The Birth of the Prison*, London: Allen Lane.

Foucault, M. (1979) *The History of Sexuality Volume 1: An Introduction*, London: Allen Lane.

Hockey, J. and James, A. (1993) *Growing Up and Growing Old: Ageing and Dependency in the Life Course*, London: Sage.

Jones, C. and Novak, T. (1999) *Poverty, Welfare and the Disciplinary State*, London: Routledge.

Millar, J. (1989) 'Social security, equality and women in the UK', *Policy and Politics*, vol. 17, no. 4.

Mishra, R. (1995) 'Social policy after socialism', in Baldock, J. and May, M. (eds) *Social Policy Review 7*: Canterbury: Social Policy Association.

Phillipson, J. (1992) *Practising Equality: Women, Men and Social Work*, London: Central Council for Education and Training in Social Work.

Rex, J. (1996) 'National identity in the democratic multi-cultural state', *Sociological Research Online*, vol. 1, no. 2, www.socresonline.org.uk/socresonline/1/2 (accessed 23 April 2001).

Righton, P. (1990) 'Orientating ourselves', Prologue to Open University K254 *Working with Children and Young People*, Milton Keynes: Open University.

Sartre, J.P. (1963) *Search for a Method*, New York: Vintage.

Small, S. (1994) *The Black Experience in the United States and England in the 1980s*, London: Routledge.

Stewart, A. (2001) *Theories of Power and Domination: The Politics of Empowerment in Late Modernity*, London: Sage.

Thompson, N. and Bates, J. (1996) *Learning From Other Disciplines*, Social Work Monograph no. 147, Norwich: University of East Anglia.

Thompson, N. (1996) *People Skills: A Guide to Effective Practice in the Human Services*, London: Macmillan.

Thompson, N. (1998a) *Promoting Equality: Challenging Discrimination and Oppression in the Human Services*, Basingstoke: Macmillan.

Thompson, N. (1998b) 'The ontology of ageing', *British Journal of Social Work*, vol. 28, no. 5.

Thompson, N. (2000a) *Theory and Practice in Human Services*, 2nd edn, Buckingham: Open University Press.

Thompson, N. (2000b) *Tackling Bullying and Harassment in the Workplace*, Birmingham, Pepar.

Thompson, N. (2001) *Anti-Discriminatory Practice*, 3rd edn, Basingstoke: Palgrave.

Thompson, S. and Thompson, N. (1993) *Perspectives on Ageing*, Social Work Monograph no. 122, Norwich: University of East Anglia.

Chapter 4

Changing agendas

Moving beyond fixed identities in anti-oppressive practice

Lena Dominelli

Introduction

Those endorsing 'New Right' philosophies have questioned the relevance of anti-oppressive approaches in social work practice. They have sought to undermine its position by arguing that it leads to politically motivated interventions that disempower the people it aims to serve (Phillips, 1993, 1994). Their critique of anti-oppressive social work has been trenchant and has had far-reaching consequences. Following from their castigation of radical practitioners and academics, British social work has undergone a series of profound changes. The Central Council for Social Work Education and Training (CCETSW) has been significantly restructured, with its Black Perspectives Committee diminished in role, and its academic chief executive replaced with a lawyer whose views of social work education have chimed in more closely with those of government in opposing social work's concerns about 'isms'. The ultimate act in this process of restructuring is the abolition of CCETSW itself, with a new body for the training and education of the profession to be established.

The attack on anti-oppressive practice has contributed to the shift of social work education away from the academy and into the workplace. This latter development has transformed the face of probation training in England and Wales where it has been de-coupled from social work education. Now, rather than trainees being provided with a university-based educational experience that equips them with both professional expertise and the capacity to critically appraise practice, probation students are required to undergo an apprenticeship that simply prepares them for 'the job'. The new probation qualification aims primarily to ensure that trainees meet the employers' requirements for National Standards of practice (Ward and Spencer, 1994; Sone, 1995). The objective of training is to enable probation officers, for example, to respond to containment objectives rather than to develop a knowledge base which has a focus on meeting offenders' needs for rehabilitation as full members of society.

This progression in probation training foreshadows the future for the social work profession more generally, particularly with regard to intensifying managerialist control over the labour process and the increased bureaucratisation of service delivery. The former is quite clear in the government's 'modernising' agenda (Department of Health, 1998), which adopts the same principles of standard setting for care management and assessment processes and procedures for the closer monitoring and inspection of those processes. The latter is evident in the emphasis on the regularity of record keeping reviews and the moves toward national standardisation of service allocation and delivery.

These developments illustrate an instrumentalist rather than an affective approach to social work education: they are overwhelmingly concerned with the efficiency of process and outcomes rather than with caring principles and the nature of human interaction. As such, they devalue the significance of both user-based and professional assessments of needs. At the same time, the approach empowers employers and managers over practitioners, users and academics in a struggle over professional knowledge expressed as who determines the nature and content of social work courses. The current outcome has also bureaucratised the character of the professional relationship between 'clients' and practitioners (Dominelli and Hoogvelt, 1996).

As a result of these changes, advocates of anti-oppressive practice are on the defensive (see Black Assessors, 1994; Dominelli, 1996). This is set against a context in which British social work at the beginning of the twenty-first century is struggling for its future as a high status, well-paid profession that can respond to the challenges set for practice by 'clients' intent on realising user-led agendas. The major focus of the debates about practice are embedded in controversies that concern the nature of professional knowledge – who should define it and how it should be disseminated to the next generation of practitioners.

In this chapter, I shall examine the controversial nature of anti-oppressive practice in the hope of clarifying its meanings and arguing that given the contemporary climate of increasing destitution and despair in this country and elsewhere (UNDP, 1998), anti-oppressive practice is needed in social work more than ever. This is particularly relevant for practice rooted in mobilising individuals and communities against poverty and injustice. I conclude that having anti-oppressive practice under siege provides an opportunity for rethinking and reconceptualising its theory and practice so that it responds more fully to user-led agendas for practice.

Defining anti-oppressive practice

'New Right' ideologues have portrayed anti-oppressive practice as a monolithic and oppressive form of intervention (Appleyard, 1993; Pinker, 1993; Phillips, 1993, 1994). However, there is no single agreed definition of anti-oppressive practice and different authors highlight particular dimensions of it. Burke and Harrison (1998: 230) define it as 'a dynamic process based on the changing complex patterns of social relations'. Braye and Preston-Shoot (1995) emphasise the importance of rooting such practice in legal frameworks that endorse equality. Clifford (1998: 65) concentrates on the interrelationship between the 'broad social structure' and its 'personal and organisational' dimensions.

In Dominelli (1994), I provide a more comprehensive definition. In it, I consider the processual nature of the interaction between the personal and structural dimensions of oppression, including that of locating the workers themselves within both the 'client'–worker relationships and their workplace settings as essential elements of this process. Additionally, I highlight the importance of: understanding the intersecting nature of the different forms of oppression that occur in any particular individual's life; advocating a holistic approach to practice because oppression touches on all points of a professional relationship – inputs, process and outcomes; identifying the need to respect its rootedness in user demands for social justice; recognising the significance of the negotiated nature of all professional interventions; considering the relevance of focusing on user agency in what are otherwise experienced as technocratic processes of intervention; and calling for practitioner proficiency of the highest order. I define anti-oppressive practice and aims as:

> a form of social welfare practice which addresses social divisions and structural inequalities in the work that is done with 'clients' (users) or workers. Anti-Oppressive Practice (AOP) aims to provide more appropriate and sensitive services by responding to people's (self-defined) needs regardless of their social status. AOP embodies: a person-centred philosophy; an egalitarian value system concerned with reducing the deleterious effects of structural inequalities upon people's lives; a methodology that focuses on both process and outcome; and a way of structuring relationships between individuals that aims to empower users by reducing the negative effects of hierarchy in their immediate interaction and work they do together.
>
> (Dominelli, 1994: 3)

These aims and definition emphasise the issue of holistically addressing personally experienced structural inequalities within the setting or context within which they occur.

Contested agendas: shifting professional concerns

Given the worthiness of the aims that practising anti-oppressive practitioners have espoused, how was it that the media and government in particular were able to subject social workers to a sustained and successful attack that peaked in the summer of 1993 by using anti-racism as its key focus? The answer to this question has a number of strands. To begin with, the profession as a whole was not convinced that social workers should be concerned with issues of oppression. The variety of positions on the issue has produced a number of fragmented discourses. These provided spaces that enabled those who lacked enthusiasm for its initiatives to eventually mount a potent attack against it. The 'New Right's' undermining of anti-oppressive practice has been achieved through the clever manipulation of rhetoric and innuendo in the press. Through this means, its critics have been able to achieve optimal effort with minimal evidence being produced to warrant taking action against anti-oppressive practice and its achievements or lack of them (see Appleyard, 1993; Pinker, 1993; Phillips, 1993, 1994). Additionally, their impact was magnified because these antagonists were powerful opinion formers who were influential in the media. Other people were more measured in their critiques. These included academics who satisfied themselves that what was at stake was the return of social work to a type of professionalism that endorsed technocratic neutrality under regimes endorsed by the status quo (see Davies, 1995).

Besides the problem of there not being a unified view of what constituted anti-oppressive practice, many of those supporting anti-oppressive stances were poorly equipped to undertake the teaching that CCETSW (1989) demanded of them under Addendum 5 of Paper 30 (Dominelli, 1997). This was the section that required social work courses to ensure an understanding of oppression and to work in anti-racist ways. A great many lecturers and practice teachers had never been trained in this area, undertaken careful study of the subject, or experienced oppression. Yet, they were suddenly forced into the position of becoming overnight experts who could both profess on these matters and assess them. The lack of training for people who possessed little basis for undertaking this teaching and the lack of mechanisms for ascertaining who was equipped to tutor others in this part of the curriculum was problematic. It resulted in individuals, whose sole qualification was a commitment towards the subject, being prevailed upon to teach it or setting themselves up as consultants having the expertise for doing so. This outcome further devalued the knowledge that went into anti-oppressive practice. However, organisations that faced the requirement to offer anti-oppressive materials and assess students according to CCETSW's standards to maintain accredited status were willing to condone such practices in the absence of other alternatives ready to hand. Consequently, examples of poor teaching and practice could be found (Jones, 1993). But, equally a number of highly successful illustrations of how to engage with this topic were available, although the media hype on the matter never reported these (see Dominelli, 1994).

At one point, CCETSW did attempt to create helpful materials under the aegis of the Northern Curriculum Development Project (NCDP) (Patel, 1994). But this endeavour drew on the expertise of a limited number of individuals selected by CCETSW and whose authority to speak on the subject was never clarified. Yet, they included academics and practitioners, 'black' and 'white', some of whom had been engaged in earlier struggles to change CCETSW's own priorities as a regulatory body supporting the status quo, and others who had not. Sadly, this grouping of people did not necessarily have credibility within the profession as a whole. Moreover, the products of their efforts were marketed as commercially viable books, with a retail price of £15 each, which meant that they were not widely purchased by those who needed them. Additionally, the merit of the materials which NCDP produced for teaching purposes was not discussed by the profession either openly or widely. Consequently, their status remained an uncertain one within which academics, students and practitioners could choose whether or not they even referred to their existence. CCETSW also appointed its own external assessors to undertake quality assurance functions, which encompassed the areas of 'race' and ethnicity, and in the process alienated key established members of the academic community. Thus, the gap between the body responsible for initiating a fundamentally important shift in what was counted as knowledge and those responsible for disseminating it through their daily practice, was widened.

Very quickly, the NCDP literature began to stand for the type of anti-oppressive approach that was being critiqued by 'New Right' ideologues and postmodernist thinkers. The former opposed its contents on ideological grounds (see Pinker, 1993). The latter group were sceptical of the CCETSW-endorsed view of what constituted anti-oppressive practice because they considered that its adherents treated each social division as homogeneous and unchanging and that, in initially focusing primarily on 'race', they ignored other important social divisions which were also significant to the 'client(s)' whom practitioners served. Although other social divisions were subsequently covered by NCDP, their analyses of the forms of discrimination to be addressed within these other areas of social division, for example in respect of disability, contained little attempt to examine the interaction between these areas, such as between disability and gender or disability and race. Consequently, postmodernists argued that anti-racists dealt with issues of 'race' and racism as reductionist and deterministic categories which had the further disadvantage of presenting 'black' people as victims of a system over which they had no control (Rojek *et al.*, 1988). This, they argued, created 'race' as an essentialist category that reified biological characteristics in ways that endorsed their being treated as both natural and immutable (Gould, 1993). Similar points were made with regard to how some anti-racists handled culture (Dominelli, 1998).

One of the difficulties in assessing the usefulness for social work of the postmodernist presentation of the issues at stake is that although the explanations provided by anti-racist and postmodernist thinkers do have different starting points and sociological concerns, both have a critically important focus on the complex areas of 'essentialism' and identity within the contemporary social order. As such, both accounts contain elements that promote our understanding of particular aspects of society and can be applied to social analysis without necessarily preferring one approach over the other. Both characterisations present a partial story that emphasises different social features. Anti-racism, as a theoretical approach, does not attempt 'grand theory': that is to say that it does not attempt to explain everything in the social order in terms of 'race'. It is more concerned with how 'race' has come to occupy and to maintain a central position in the development of welfare and to rectify racial injustice. In this respect it shares certain features with postmodernism, which is much concerned with the origins of knowledge and power, and with examining how different aspects of a particular social order come to be explained in public discourses in the way that they are.

Anti-racism appropriately highlights a way of defining 'race' that is reflected in racist ideology, where 'race', as represented in ordinary discourses among people, is both essentialised and socially constructed. Racism in popular culture is the expression of social relations organised on the basis of the imputed superiority of one 'race' over another, the presumption being that the allegedly superior 'race' can dominate or oppress the others (Dominelli, 1988). In racist paradigms, 'race' is essentialised into an immutable category to justify social relations that endorse racism and privilege 'white' people. This representation of the situation enables those who consider themselves racially superior to act as 'subjects' entitled to treat those they consider inferior as 'objects' in every interaction with them, and thereby to exercise their agency.

In racialised discourses, this subject/object dichotomy presupposes a biological basis to differences between peoples that can be socially constructed as signifiers of 'difference' (Hall and Du Gay, 1996; Hall, 1997), imputing inferiority to that which is standing outside normalised 'whiteness'. This belief is used to organise social relations in ways that create a racialised hierarchy that privileges 'whiteness' by having 'white' people with light skin, blonde hair and blue eyes at its apex, while 'black' people with black skin, black hair and black eyes are at the bottom.

For postmodernists the representation of 'race' in these discourses is inadequate. It is considered reductionist, crude and homogenised, and as a category lacking in analysis of process and appreciation of the way that meanings about 'race' are negotiated. They point out that 'race' has variable meanings that depend on context. At the same time, postmodern analyses have failed to deal with historical continuities and systemic patterns of

oppression that impact upon the life circumstances of any particular grouping regardless of the extent to which an individual may feel that such a
categorisation does or does not fit with their experience.

For example, the discourses through which racialised hierarchies are
(re)created contain both continuities and discontinuities as particular
refrains are (re)affirmed and then modified over time. Changes occur according to how discourses are (re)framed by different actors as these are (re)pro-
duced through routine interactions in specific situations aimed at meeting
particular goals. In turn, the dynamics of everyday oppression (Essed, 1991)
are shaped by individuals or groups deciding to accept, ignore or challenge
racialised hierarchies of domination.

Social workers use traditional unitary views of identity when they focus on
shared characteristics between and among people. In these, they act upon
assumptions evident in much of the human development literature (see
Erikson, 1965, 1968) that portrays identity formation as complete once the
mature status of adulthood has been achieved. Hence, in this sense, identity
is conceptualised as a singular, fixed process that has a natural closure as it
proceeds in a linear manner over time from birth to death. In focusing on
unity, this portrayal of identity has obliterated difference, even though this
might not have reflected the specific reality of the individuals they have
been working with or even the intentions of the practitioners themselves.
This outcome is precipitated whether or not they espouse anti-oppressive
values. For being committed to these in the abstract, enables equality to
become elided into sameness. That is, everyone is the same – a part of a
homogeneous whole in which a unitary national identity is rooted. Lorenz
(1994) argues that equating equality with sameness is politically (in its
general sense) motivated, for these practitioners have been driven to relate
to identity as a unitary entity by the more general process of establishing a
national identity and their own professional space within the nation-state.
Treating 'black' people the same as 'white' people or all women the same
as men or each other are illustrative of such practice.

Reconceptualising identity for anti-oppressive practice

A central problem in addressing the issue of identity within anti-oppressive
discourses relating to 'race', was the failure of those belonging to the dominant social group to see themselves as racialised beings – a point I initially
raised in 1988 and which was subsequently theorised more substantially by
others. The key message here was that 'whiteness' could not be excluded
from being interrogated as a racialised category. Not acknowledging being
'white', as part of a process of racialising others that involves the externalis-
ing and ascribing of racial attributes to those who are different from the
'white' person, colludes with racist characterisations of 'race' and prolongs

the privileging of 'whiteness' in discussions about 'race' (Delgado and Stefancic, 1997; Frankenburg, 1997; Kincheloe *et al.*, 2000). Rather than neglecting this issue, these authors have 'demanded that whiteness' come under scrutiny too. The creation of a privileged 'gaze' centred on 'whiteness' established a dyadic hierarchical relationship between the categories 'black' and 'white'. In these relationships, 'white' is deemed superior (Dominelli, forthcoming) and outside the frame of reference that applies to the racialised 'other' who is deemed inferior. Similar points can be made about the mainstream 'gaze' on any other social division, where the dominant part of the dyad within which identities are constructed is privileged at the expense of the one deemed subordinate. So, 'women' are (re)cast as inferior to 'men' and so on. At the same time, everyone is implicated in creating 'the gaze', whether it is to reproduce dominant versions of it, challenge it from a marginalised position, or seek to create alternatives to it.

In dominant discourses, racialised hierarchies are embedded in relations of domination and foster white supremacy. These privilege 'whiteness' and create white people as 'subjects' who can ignore 'race' in the formation of their own identity as racialised (usually unacknowledged) 'subjects'. This allows for the externalisation of 'race' issues as matters that concern 'the other', or the racialised 'object' who can be oppressed on the basis of 'race' with little further thought being given to the specifics of the interaction between the two parties. In social work, this was typical of 'universalist' approaches to 'clients'. These obliterated differences between individual 'clients' and assumed that since all 'clients' were at the same starting point, their needs for help were the same and could be met from the same resources that had been set up to deal with the problems experienced by 'clients' from the dominant group. Consequently, practice regimes utilised in the UK among 'white', 'black' or working-class 'clients' were transported overseas and applied in the treatment of 'indigenous' peoples. The relevance of paradigms for practice rooted in valuing 'white' English middle-class culture and its imputed superior status in the world was not questioned, but assumed appropriate (see Haig-Brown, 1988; Bruyere, 2001; Tait-Rolleston and Pehi-Barlow, 2001). And, in the process of treating others according to its precepts, the unique personal and group identity of the specific person(s) being treated as the object(s) of their ministrations was obliterated.

These responses typify a further shortcoming that postmodernists have identified: anti-oppressive social workers' inadequate treatment of identity, whether it related to the person who oppressed others or those who were oppressed. Caution has to be exercised in considering this stance, for it does not take account of the diversity of positions that exist among anti-oppressive practitioners and analysts, and their own dynamism and variability over time. For example, Price (1996) identifies the importance of focusing on the complexities of identity experienced by disabled women in order to provide services that meet their needs. I argue that oppression strikes at the heart of 'who we are' – how we perceive ourselves, and how others define us, and, in doing so, brings issues of identity to the fore in anti-oppressive practice (Dominelli, forthcoming). I also consider identity as an interactive process that requires the self-concept of those labelled 'oppressors' to be examined and deconstructed to the same extent as that of those deemed 'oppressed' (Dominelli, 2000b). Additionally, both categories need to be understood in terms of their intellectual content along-side the feelings that they arouse in both the oppressor and the oppressed, regardless of the criteria used to differentiate one person or group from the other. Identity formation, therefore, is an interactive process that consti-tutes who we are individually and collectively. In this, different social divisions are constituted simultaneously to create a multifaceted, multi-dimensional self (Dominelli, forthcoming).

In addition to acknowledging the ways in which postmodernist critiques draw our attention to critical problems inherent in the concept of identity, those seeking to develop anti-oppressive practice themselves have voiced other related concerns. One of these has been the tendency of a number of those endorsing anti-oppressive practice to treat it as a purely intellectual project. Students, for example, have been expected simply to learn a checklist or toolkit intended to equip them to practice in anti-oppressive ways. This approach has been criticised for ignoring the complex interaction between the hand, head and heart (the 3Hs) (Dominelli, 1994). This can be reframed as the integration of practice skills, intellectual understanding and emotional capacities of the individual practitioner in interaction with those of the 'client'. Bringing these three components together in a relationship requires the exercise of critical judgement and a considerable degree of self-knowledge if the practitioner is to probe sensitively and effectively into a person's life-story and acquire a detailed knowledge of the other person (or group), with regard to those aspects of identity that impinge upon their professional interaction with one another. I have called this relational contextualisation of (1) practice skills, (2) intellectual understanding and (3) emotional capacity (including empathy), the PIE triangle for understanding oppression (Dominelli, 2000b).

Acting within this complex understanding of the integration of theory and practice demands that practitioners understand the concept of 'othering'. The dynamics of oppression are closely linked to othering processes that reproduce the antagonistic 'them–us' division in social relationships to reinforce exclusion in particular situations. I have defined 'othering' as:

> an active process of interaction that relies on the creation and re-creation of dyadic social relations in which one group is socially dominant and others are socially subordinate. In the case of racialised 'othering', physical or cultural attributes are created as signifiers of inferiority through the organisation of social relations that establish

this dyadic relationship as the context within which an encounter perpetuates the domination of one group by another.

(Dominelli, 2000c: 143)

Consequently, relations of domination are reproduced during interactions that 'other' those involved in them, and thereby construct the dominant individual (or group) in the relationship as 'subject' and the oppressed one(s) as 'object'. In contrast, egalitarian relations can exist only when both parties to an encounter can act as 'subjects' and treat each other as such. Doing so requires them to acknowledge the existence of differentiated power relations between them and create the basis for a negotiated power relationship.

'Othering' also involves practitioners in policing the boundaries of social behaviour. Key to this process is the policing of state, civil society and household boundaries. The state, through legislative fiat and the employment of regulatory personnel which include those working in the 'social' professions, has a central part to play in the process. Social workers express their role in the policing of these boundaries through their controlling activities. The boundaries between these three spheres are overlapping and change over time and according to context, but they deal with specific dimensions of social life. State boundaries are patrolled through regulations and the specification of rights, one of which is to identify entitlement (or not) to services by particular groups or individuals. At this point, creating the myth of a homogeneous national entity assists in rationing resources by excluding those popularly deemed not to *belong* to it. The boundaries of civil society are controlled through normative injunctions based upon an etiquette that defines what constitutes (non)acceptable behaviour, a set of obligations or duties towards others which may be reciprocated at least among those accepted as living within a particular polity and solidarity whereby communities of support, however transitory, are established. The household or domestic sphere is bounded by a particular version of morality and responsibilities that govern intimate relationships and define a tight circle within which life is carried out.

Both minority and majority 'gazes' interact with these boundaries to create social relationships with those (un)like them. In other words, neither oppressor nor oppressed persons can exist on their own, they are both participants in the process of creating and maintaining these statuses. That is why, from an oppressing person's point of view, it is crucial to engage the oppressed person in policing their own boundaries through consensual acts that endorse their particular version of reality or principles for defining and organising it. Equally, recognition of this dynamic of oppression enables subjugated people to break away from the prevailing consensus, form alternative visions of society and set about their realisation.

Challenging the status quo is not simply the prerogative of oppressed persons. Given that doing so requires the exercise of agency, an oppressing individual may also choose to question the unwarranted privileging of his or her own existence. Acknowledging and critiquing the exploitative basis of their hegemonic position in their interaction with others is essential to the process of moving outside of their privileged status and seeking other ways of relating to those individuals who are not from their own (dominant) group.

Within 'othering' frameworks, power relations are understood as 'power over' relations in which the group that has power exercises it over those that do not. The power to define what constitutes valued or devalued identities in this version of reality lies in the hands of the dominant group who then prescribe the common basis for identity and expect others, particularly those employed in the state apparatus, to accept and perpetuate their work. In short, these powerholders are engaged in a zero-sum game that does not acknowledge other people as anything other than 'objects' that they can manipulate to maintain their privileged position. The execution of these dynamics can be either explicit or implicit. Constituting them to affirm taken-for-granted realities in the human condition is an important aspect of the dynamics that enable these inegalitarian power relations to remain implicit and thereby more easily reproduced unintentionally. Social workers employing a 'colourblind' approach towards 'race' signify this situation.

In addition, within a context of fixed identities, social workers looking for certainties in an uncertain world, are likely to focus on one aspect of identity at the expense of other equally important dimensions, and thus miss out on the intersecting nature of different social divisions along which oppression can occur. Or, if social workers do acknowledge these, they tend to be 'added on' to an initial inadequate analytical framework. Moreover, they consider 'difference' as inferior, a deficit that has to be made good, and it reinforces attitudes that suggest, 'I'm OK, you're not OK' types of relationship. Values are deemed absolute and other people are cast as passive individuals who operate within fixed relationships and given contexts.

In contrast to this, postmodernists focus on the diverse characteristics that go into making up any one particular person. Identity is seen as a fluid formation, always in the process of becoming rather than one with an end product. Acknowledging the changing nature of identity formation and the cultures within which it is formed has led to a cultural relativism in which all cultures are considered equal and power as being shared (see Lum, 2000). Inclusion and acceptance of difference are key features in this milieu (Nicholson, 1990). However, when measured against 'client' demands, this characterisation of the situation is problematic. Cultures are not simply relative. Power relations exist within and between cultures, resulting in some being valued more than others. Moreover, cultures have both continuities and discontinuities that can be traced over time and in different geographical locations, as Brah's (1997) work on cartographies of diaspora indicates.

People can demonstrate in both their individual lifestories, and collective ones, features that persist over time and space as well as modifications that respond to changing circumstances. Looking at identities in terms of continuities and discontinuities that are dynamically reproduced through negotiated interactions between people would enable social workers to appreciate both strands of the matter. Then, instead of looking for a 'toolkit' for each culture that they proceed to apply uncritically to all people whom they deem belong to a specific culture, they can engage in more sensitive and appropriate assessments. These would be based not on stereotypes but on the specific meaning of any culture for a particular individual at a given point in time (Dominelli, 1998).

For those working in anti-oppressive ways, I advocate the conceptualisation of identities as fluid and situational. No one person's identity is lived as a fragmented entity with clear divisions among its different component parts. For example, an older disabled gay 'black' man of Jamaican origin living in England would experience all these modalities of existence at any one point in time. However, he might emphasise different aspects of his identity, depending on the goal or purpose of a particular relationship. So, for example, in a gay club, he might focus on his sexual orientation. But, if asking for a personal social service, he might want the social worker to respond to him as a whole being with particular needs.

Grounding their interventions within fluid identities and holistic client-centred approaches, anti-oppressive practitioners would focus on the strengths of those they encounter and act to value and celebrate 'difference' in a situational context that advocates human rights and recognises people as active agents. Process issues would also be appreciated as dynamic and interactive. And, as relationships would be conceptualised as revolving around negotiations with others, power would be experienced as constantly being created and recreated. Thus, power would be expressed as a multifaceted and multidimensional phenomenon and not a zero-sum game. Individuals would be seen as having a degree of choice about the lifestyles they choose to lead without losing track of the structural dimensions within which their choices are embedded.

To promote a holistic anti-oppressive practice, social workers constantly have to examine the work they do with their 'clients' and reflect critically upon their own practice. This includes recognising that they are engaged in a relationship, however brief, with another person. At the same time, it involves accepting that there is an interaction between the practitioner's sense of self, position in society and view of the other person alongside the 'client's' sense of self, life circumstances and perceptions of the practitioner. It also means that practitioners have to focus on making a holistic appraisal of the situation by focusing on the basis of their assessment, the nature of their relationship with their 'client' and the 'client's' position with regard to their broader social and physical environments. Alongside their inter-action with one another, this has to include the linking of theory and practice, their handling of issues of oppression along all relevant social dimensions, and using research findings to ensure that they are aware of significant materials in their field.

The recognition of identity as a central feature in interpersonal relation-ships indicates the extent to which some postmodernist thinkers have similar concerns to those of anti-oppressive theorists. However, there is a key dis-tinction to be drawn between the two approaches in respect of the creation of more appropriate forms of social welfare practice. This is the advocacy within anti-oppressive theory of collective action as a basis for social change and the transformation of those social structures that adversely shape individual choices and life opportunities.

Key principles that underpin the holistic approach of anti-oppressive social work include the following: social justice; rights and citizenship; solidarity; reciprocity and interdependence; and valuing strengths (Domi-nelli, forthcoming). Social justice is a value that promotes equality in matters of power and resource distribution. It is also about ensuring that a person is treated with dignity and respect. The idea of rights locates an individual or group within a set of social relationships in which they have access to and receive social and material resources as inalienable entitlements when needed. This is particularly important in moving social work out of its stig-matised status and getting rid of its image as a charitable institution that is dependent on personal discretion and goodwill towards others. Citizenship is closely allied to the possession of rights, although in the current conjunc-ture, with mass migrations of people from one part of the world to another, for citizenship to be an inclusive rather than an exclusive category (Lister, 1997), it needs to encompass the notion of global citizenship (Dominelli, 1997). It has to transcend national borders and requires new instruments for administration (Dominelli, 2000b).

Solidarity embraces the realisation of the value of supporting others through the formation of mutual links of collaboration and support net-works. Solidarity is crucial because it provides the basis both for establishing reciprocal relationships and for acknowledging the interdependent nature of social relations. Reciprocity is the acknowledgement of both giving and receiving when interacting with others to obtain assistance. Interdependence involves the realisation that no person or group is sufficient unto them-selves. There are relational ties that bind diverse peoples to each other, even when they are not directly in contact with each other, as long as no one person can meet all of his or her own needs entirely on his or her own. Interdependence can be seen as underpinning all of the other features that contribute to the development of more egalitarian relationships between practitioners and 'clients'.

Conclusion

Challenging oppression in relation to key issues such as poverty and social marginalisation that underpin interactions in social welfare requires a holistic approach to social change that tackles oppression at the personal, institutional and cultural levels. It involves practitioners and educators locating themselves in relations aimed at countering oppression, since a person can be both oppressing as well as oppressed, depending on which particular features and social positions are at issue. Social change requires the mobilisation of collective energies and the creation of networks of solidarity in which people interact with each other as 'subjects'. Identity formation must be seen as a complex and contested process in which different actors play different roles. These may include those of hanging on to privileges that are accrued through the enactment of unequal social relations just as much as roles in which struggles to overturn these privileges, in the interests of social justice and solidarity, are pursued. Anti-oppressive practice that is allowed to flower in the work that is done with individuals or groups is well placed to promote egalitarian relations in and through social work. It is time to move it away from the state of siege that keeps social work marginalised and prevents it from realising its potential to contribute to the liberation of peoples.

References

Appleyard, B. (1993) 'Why paint so black a picture', in *The Independent*, 4 August.

Black Assessors (1994) 'DipSW Consultations a Sham', *Community Care*, 13–18 October.

Brah, A. (1997) *Cartographies of Diaspora: Contesting Identities – Gender, Racism and Ethnicity*, London: Routledge.

Braye, S. and Preston-Shoot, M. (1995) *Empowering Practice in Social Care*, Buckingham: Open University Press.

Burke, B. and Harrison, P. (1998) 'Anti-Oppressive Practice', in Adams, R., Dominelli, L. and Payne, M. (eds) *Social Work: Themes, Issues and Current Debates*, London: Macmillan.

Bruyere, G. (2001) 'Making circles: renewing first nations ways of helping', in Dominelli, L., Lorenz, W. and Soydan, H. (eds), *Beyond Racial Divides: Ethnicities in Social Work*, Aldershot: Ashgate.

Central Council for Education and Training in Social Work (CCETSW) Requirements and Regulations for the Diploma in Social Work, revised 1991 and 1995, London: CCETSW.

Clifford, D. (1998) *Social Assessment Theory and Practice*, Aldershot: Ashgate.

Davies, M. (1995) *The Essential Social Worker: A Guide to Positive Practice*, Aldershot: Gower.

Delgado, R. and Stefancic, J. (eds) (1997) *Critical White Studies: Looking Behind the Mirror*, Philadelphia: Temple University Press.

Department of Health (1998) *Modernising Social Services: Promoting Independence, Improving Protection, Raising Standards*, London: Stationery Office.

Dominelli, L. (1988) *Anti-Racist Social Work,* London: Macmillan.

Dominelli, L. (1994) 'Models of Anti-Racist Education', in Dominelli, L., Patel, N. and Thomas Bernard, W. (eds) *Anti-Racist Social Work Education*, Sheffield: Department of Sociological Studies, University of Sheffield.

Dominelli, L. (1996) 'Deprofessionalising Social Work: Anti-Oppressive Practice, Competencies and Postmodernism', *British Journal of Social Work*, vol. 26.

Dominelli, L. (1997) *Sociology for Social Work*, London: Macmillan.

Dominelli, L. (1998) *Critiquing Culturally Competent Approaches to Social Work*, Paper delivered to the CSWE Anti-Racist Task Force, 4 December, Ann Arbor: University of Michigan.

Dominelli, L. (2000a) *Global Citizenship: Pipe Dream or Reality?*, Paper given at the CIAC Annual Conference, 6 June, Montreal.

Dominelli, L. (2000b) *Partnerships in Child Welfare Practice: The Field, the Academy and 'Clients' Relating Together in the 'Multiversity'*, Paper given at the Annual Lecture of Swedish Social Workers, 24 November, Stockholm, Sweden.

Dominelli, L. (2000c) 'Tackling Racism in Everyday Realities: A Task for Social Workers', in Callahan, M. and Hessle, S. (eds) *Valuing the Field: Child Welfare in an International Context*, Aldershot: Ashgate.

Dominelli, L. (forthcoming) *Anti-Oppressive Practice: From Oppressive to Empowering Social Work*, London: Palgrave.

Dominelli, L. and Hoogvelt, A. (1996) 'The Technocratisation of Social Work', *Critical Social Policy*, vol. 47, no. 2.

Erikson, E. (1965) *Childhood and Society*, Harmondsworth: Penguin.

Erikson, H. (1968) *Identity, Youth and Crisis*, London: Faber.

Essed, P. (1991) *Everyday Racism: Report from Women of Two Cultures*, New York: Hunter House.

Frankenburg, R. (1997) *Displacing Whiteness: Essays in Social and Cultural Criticism*, Durham, NC: Duke University Press.

Gould, N. (1993) 'Anti-Racist Social Work: A Framework for Teaching and Action', *Issues in Social Work Education*, vol. 14, no.1.

Haig-Brown, C. (1988) *Resistance and Renewal: Surviving the Indian Residential School*, Vancouver: Tillicum Library and Arsenal Pulp Press.

Hall, S. (1997) *Representation: Cultural Representation and Signifying Practices: Culture, Media and Identity, Volume 2*, London: Sage.

Hall, S. and Du Gay, P. (1996) *Questions of Cultural Identity*, London: Sage.

Jones, C. (1993) 'Distortion and Demonisation: The Right and Anti-Racist Social Work Education', *Social Work Education*, vol. 12, no. 12.

Kincheloe, J., Steinberg, S.R., Rodriquez, N. and Chennault, R.S. (eds) (2000) *White Reign: Displacing Whiteness in America*, London: Palgrave.

Lister, R. (1997) *Citizenship: A Feminist Perspective*, London: Macmillan.

Lorenz, W. (1994) *Social Work in a Changing Europe*, New York: Routledge.

Lum, D. (2000) *Culturally Competent Practice: A Framework for Growth and Action*, Pacific Grove, CA: Brooks/Cole Publishing.

Nicholson, L. (1990) *Postmodernism/Feminism*, London: Routledge.

Patel, N. (1994) 'CCETSW', in Dominelli, L., Patel, N. and Thomas Bernard, W. (eds) *Anti-Racist Social Work Education*, Sheffield: Department of Sociological Studies, University of Sheffield.

Phillips, M. (1993) 'An Oppressive Urge to End Oppression', *The Observer*, 1 August.

Phillips, M. (1994) 'Illiberal Liberalism', in Dunant, S. (ed.) *The War of the Words: The Political Correctness Debate*, London: Virago.

Pinker, R. (1993) 'A Lethal Kind of Looniness', *The Times Higher Educational Supplement*, 10 September.

Price, J. (1996) 'The Marginal Politics of Our Bodies: Women's Health, the Disability Movement and Power', in Humphries, B. (ed.) *Critical Perspectives on Empowerment*, Birmingham: Venture Press.

Rojek, C., Peacock, G. and Collins, S. (1988) *Social Work and Received Ideas*, London: Routledge.

Sone, K. (1995) 'Get Tough', *Community Care*, 16-22 March, pp. 16–18.

Tait-Rolleston, W. and Pehi-Barlow, S. (2001) 'A Maori Social Work Construct', in Dominelli, L., Lorenz, W. and Soydan, H. (eds), *Beyond Racial Divides: Ethnicities in Social Work*, Aldershot: Ashgate.

United Nations Development Programme (UNDP) (1998) *Human Development, 2000*, New York: UNDP.

Ward, D. and Spencer, J. (1994) 'The Future of Probation Qualifying Training', *Probation Journal*, 41(2).

Chapter 5

The political challenge of anti-racism in social care and health

Gurnam Singh

Introduction

This chapter is divided into three sections. The first section sets out a theoretical and historical argument for understanding contemporary racism and anti-racism. In particular, I point to some of the problems with a form of identity politics that has a tendency to both factionalise anti-racism and to de-couple it from other struggles against oppression such as those around disability, class, gender and sexuality. The second section examines some of the current debates surrounding the issue of institutionalised racism and considers whether the Macpherson Report (1999) has anything new to offer towards the struggle against racism. The chapter concludes by setting out some principles for the further development of anti-racist and anti-oppressive practice within health and welfare services.

The roots of racist ideology

In beginning to prepare this chapter, and being very conscious to focus on a 'way forward', it was clearly incumbent on me to specify the location of the current position, and this, in turn, required knowledge of how that location had been reached. In this respect, I suggest that it is only through a critical examination of our historical trajectory that we can begin to discern the scope and relevance of any proposed future actions. In taking such an approach, and notwithstanding the problems of historicism posed by post-structuralists like Foucault, I soon became aware of other problems of relativism which are an inevitable part of endeavours such as this. Where does the past begin? Hall (1992) notes that the most interesting thing about the past is not the date of any particular event but where and why we draw lines at certain points. For example, there is now general consensus among anthropologists that Africa is indeed the birthplace of *Homo sapiens*, but I guess that not all readers of this volume would, for an innumerable variety of reasons, not necessarily wish to claim a share of African ancestry. And so a critical question to ask is: 'what are the ideological, social and political points of intersection and rupture that shape the social world and our percep-tions of it?'

In relation to the contemporary debates about race and ethnicity I guess 1492 is one such point of rupture. As is well known, this is the year that the Genoese explorer Christopher Columbus sailed from the Iberian penin-sula to seek a new route to India by sailing westward. Unhappily for his purpose, he 'bumped' into the Caribbean islands, which he called the West Indies. Though less well known, another important event that has much reso-nance with the recent events in the Balkans, happened in Spain in the same year. Almost the entire Muslim majority of Spain was deported from their homeland, many of them ending up in the Balkans, the scene of so much tragedy and violence in recent times. It is also around this period that the beginnings of the racialisation process can be identified, a process resulting in the eventual division of the globe into these spurious things called 'nations' and 'races'.

Of equal importance with these cultural and racial 'turning points' in history, as Williams (1996) asserts in his discussion of capitalism and slavery, from the end of the sixteenth century onwards we are beginning to see the large-scale exploitation of human labour for the accumulation of capital. Indeed, contrary to popular belief, it is probably Columbus rather than Bill Gates who is really responsible for what we know as the process of 'globalisation'.

Binary oppositions and identity formation

What have all these excursions into history to do with anti-racist practice and anti-oppressive practice? Quite simply, in order to begin to conceptualise anti-racism, it is first necessary to understand the intricate meshing of racist ideology with coercive force and capital over the past five hundred years.

What makes racist ideology particularly difficult to identify is that it often operates by stealth. Through the use of prevailing dominant discourses, such as those of science and professionalism, racist ideology constantly seeks to obscure and naturalise relations of dominance. Language and the operation of binary oppositions plays a critical function in this process. Derrida (1978) in particular offers an understanding of how the development of binary oppositions performs a key function in the construction of dominant and subjugated identities within Western culture. Thus concepts such as rational/irrational, good/evil, white/black, man/woman, straight/gay, objec-tive/subjective, moral/immoral, modern/primitive, etc., in which the first is regarded as superior and the second a threat to it, play a critical role in the production and reproduction of oppression.

One of the central preoccupations of both racist and anti-racist discourse is the struggle over 'identity'. Rattansi suggests that the only way to conceive the various forms of Western racism is to understand the centrality of the notion of identity to the production and reproduction of racism. He states that:

> 'Western' identities – and those of its Others – have continually been formed and created by actual and imagined encounters with the non-Western Others of modernity. Identities such as 'the West', 'European', and 'white'.

(Rattansi, 1994: 36)

It is through the conflation of these identities with conceptions of rationality and 'civilisation', and the superimposition upon these images of paganism and savagery as constituted by binarisms such as naked/clothed, oral/literate, primitive/advanced and so on, that racism is reproduced. In other words, racism becomes understood not merely as an ideology for the justification and legitimisation of oppression, but much more profoundly as a philosophy of history, depicted as a process of struggle between 'stronger' more 'gifted' 'races' and 'weaker' 'races'.

The paradox of identity

The struggle over identity has historically constituted a key dimension of anti-racist struggle. From demands for ethnically sensitive service provision to heated debates about same 'race' placements for black children in care, the pull of identity based politics and practice is indeed strong.

However, a particular notion of identity, as being unified, with corporeal properties forms a key paradox that has, in the past, confronted anti-racism and continues to prove problematic today. A common-sense view might be that a clear sense of identity allows us to answer such questions as: 'who we are?', 'where we belong?' and 'where did we come from?' However, a closer examination of identity reveals it as complex, often contradictory, fragmented, multiple, and in a constant state of flux. The 'real' self is nowhere to be found other than in our daily encounters with each other.

Let me illustrate this point with a personal example. Some fifteen years ago at the age of twenty-five I returned to India for the first time since my early childhood, having been brought up in the UK from the age of two. I went with the full expectation that my identity as an Indian would be confirmed. But to my surprise, to Indians resident in India I was a 'blety' (derived from the word blighty), or a 'Britisher'. Reference was even made to my 'fair skin'. Not only was this difference held to be significant, but I also felt that Indians believed me to be superior in many respects and showed great deference towards me. From my own personal point of view, the worst aspect of the encounter was, that from leaving England with a very certain sense of my 'Indianness', for the first time in my life I felt like an Englishman and, to my shame, I even felt superior because of it! The experience illustrates quite graphically that there is nothing intrinsic about self-identity, but that it is always produced in the social and cultural sphere; very often mediated through unequal power relations.

On the one hand we seem to have a deep desire for believing in the notion of a true identity, hidden within the deep crevices of our being. There is something very appealing and reassuring about this idea. Not only does it help us, as Hall (1992) suggests, to sleep well at night, it also helps us to negotiate the many discontinuities and ruptures of society. Our identity becomes a kind of refuge, or bunker from which to negotiate the other.

Yet, on the other hand, the desire for a strong uncritically held sense of 'ethnic' or 'racial' identity can lead to racism. Take for example the horrific acts of the so called 'ethnic' cleansing in the former Yugoslavia, or the unfolding tragedy in Indonesia. When, during the long-running Tory administration of the 1980s and 1990s, the then government Minister Norman Tebbit posed the 'cricket test' and the then Prime Minister Margaret Thatcher expressed the fear of 'swamping', and when successive Home Secretaries acted to further bolster the immigration and nationality laws (*Daily Mail*, 31 January 1978; Solomos, 1989), each in their own way was addressing a spurious ethnic identity. This identity is never exactly defined, but it is one which, in conceptual terms is perfectly real, as Darcus Howe's notion of 'the White Tribe' suggests (Channel 4, January–February 2000).

When the assailants of Stephen Lawrence decided to target and then kill him, they too could be seen, in this respect, to be acting upon some secure sense of their own and Stephen's identity and difference. If it is argued that Stephen's killers were not born racists, then it can only be concluded that the antecedents of their murderous racist behaviour must have been the material and discursive dimensions of the society in which they were socialised. Thus they too can be understood as products of institutional and structural racism. Nonetheless, as Thompson points out in Chapter 3 of this volume, there is a widespread tendency in British society to regard racism as primarily something perpetuated by a small minority of ill-educated and prejudiced individuals. It is easier for the society as a whole if these individuals are strongly dealt with as 'animals' and as representing a stain on the character of an otherwise non-racist nation. In the same way, placing the blame for racism in the police force on a few corrupt officers of the 'Met' leaves the rest of the force unscathed.

From Scarman to Macpherson

In 1981, following a summer of inner-city riots, an independent judicial enquiry by Lord Scarman issued a report on 'race' and policing in the UK. As part of the establishment concerns associated with this report and the earlier 1976 Race Relations Act, the 'race relations industry' was given birth, with its all too familiar and disappointing outcomes. While perhaps opening up career opportunities for a small number of black people as professionals, providing racism awareness training and funding the construction of community centres, very little inroad was made into the structural and endemic aspects of racism.

Eighteen years later another report was issued. Again, the focus was on policing and black people. This time it was the turn of Lord Macpherson, who, in a way that Scarman did not, was able to articulate in a much more precise way the complex functioning of institutionalised racism. In contrast to Scarman's emphasis on the individual prejudiced behaviour of some police officers, Macpherson (1999: Section 6.34) rightly placed the responsibility on 'the collective failure of an organisation to provide an appropriate and professional service to people because of their colour, culture, or ethnic origin'.

In interrogating not only the experiences of black people but also the workings of the Metropolitan Police Force, Macpherson found that while the experience of racism can be very brutal, its workings are very often extremely subtle, hidden and more pervasive and endemic than was ever imagined by Scarman. Moreover, in recommending that all public bodies should be subject to the Race Relations Act, clearly Macpherson presented policy makers and practitioners with an unprecedented challenge.

Despite the welcome given to Macpherson by the then Home Secretary, Jack Straw, it was noteworthy that, in the introduction of the new Race Relations Bill during the Queen's speech of 17 November 1999, it was proposed only to extend it to the police and other governmental bodies in relation to *direct* discrimination. Straw's defence in leaving out indirect discrimination seems to have been that the government would not be able to function under a hail of potential lawsuits; which seems to be an admission that the state is racist and nothing can be done about it. But then perhaps, the whole Stephen Lawrence case says more about the insatiable desire of the media for sensational stories and spin doctors, than about any serious desire to create a just and equal society.

Current situation: where do we go next?

First, all of those working in health and welfare areas, as part of their commitment to anti-racism, can deploy Macpherson in the same way that Scarman was deployed. While Scarman was helpful in drawing attention to the problems which black and white youth alike faced in their relations with the police, Macpherson is of course of most value in drawing attention to the prevalence of institutional racism. Prior to Macpherson, progressive anti-racists drawing attention to endemic and institutional racism were being dismissed as the lunatic fringe and/or naïve peddlers of political correctness.

All those who have responsibilities in health, social and other welfare services can now take strength from Macpherson and begin to exert pressure for change in the specific policies, practices and procedures of their own organisations. Organisations are of course a microcosm of society, and thus the wider struggles against state sponsored racism, against the asylum, immigration and nationality laws, against deaths in police custody, against stop and search, against racism in the judicial system, against school exclusions, against the premature deaths of black people due to health inequalities, and against the economic policies leading to the devastation of the inner cities where the vast majority of black people live are always relevant to worker–client interactions. The recent debate on the 'north–south divide' failed to mention that a key economic divide is between black and white. As Sivanandan (2000) suggests, 'in the final analysis, institutional racism is the litmus test of a society's democracy'.

Developing anti-racist/anti-oppressive practice

Political/ideological perspectives

In terms of politics and ideology, I suggest that a strategy for anti-racist/ anti-oppressive practice can be set out as follows:

1 Connect the material and discursive dimensions of racism. The emphasis on this connection is based on an understanding that discursive formations are critical because it is these that often act to reinforce, contradict, conceal, explain or 'explain away' the materiality or history of any given situation (Frankenberg, 1993). It is the meshing of discursive repertoires with material reality that gives rise to 'experience' and political cause. Take for example the experience of black people in the mental health or criminal justice system. Clearly, without an understanding of the complex meshing of colonial and slave discourses, and the idea and practice of incarceration of deviant populations within Western industrial societies, one cannot even begin to dismantle these systems of oppression.

2 Develop a relationship between human suffering as it is manifest in the problems of clients, on the one hand, and on the other as it is presented as an observable product of systems of dominance. This, in turn requires us to seek out the intersections between racism, sexism, homophobia, disablism, ageism, classism or indeed all distortions of difference that may produce stigma and oppression.

3 Realise that the celebration of difference is a double-edged sword and refuse to deny the potential significance of difference while at the same time not assuming that difference is all pervasive. As human beings we have much more in common with each other than not.

4   Oppose the separation of populations on the basis of essentialist constructions of 'race', ethnicity, nation, religion, etc.

5   Actively resist social control and coercive measures against targeted populations, for example refugees and asylum seekers.

6   Provide for integrative services and commitment to principles of self-help and community development

7   Move beyond the black/white binarism and develop a much more inclusive anti-racist movement, for example by including Irish, Jewish, Muslim, Roma, and East European refugee populations.

8   Link anti-racist demands much more closely to a human rights, civil rights and social justice agenda and other struggles against oppression.

Professional practice perspectives

In terms of profession-defined areas of activity, I suggest that anti-racist/anti-oppressive practice can be developed if we are mindful of the following principles:

1   Anti-oppressive practice (AOP) involves workers recognising the power that they hold both in terms of representing an agency with its many resources, and as individuals, due to such advantages as their often holding middle-class status, being white, young or middle-aged and able-bodied. It is also important to take note of power deriving from personal skills. Whatever health and social service workers' intentions may be, it cannot be assumed that because of their over-riding 'helping' objective, everything done is beneficial to the client group. Professionalism is a process which rarely takes account of the ways in which workers are, to varying degrees, responsible for carrying out the policies which result in oppression. The part which professionals play in oppression has always to be borne in mind, as does the fact that it is too often the case that they choose not to do anything to challenge oppression.

2   AOP involves learning to identify the ideas (of self, of others and of institutions) and processes which contribute to oppression. This can be achieved by, for example, education in the fields of health and social service which enables students to evaluate the stereotypes and myths about the superiority of European civilisation and British culture that are learned through overt and covert socialisation processes, and by their learning about the history of racism and oppression and the origins of the deep-rooted, distorted ideas and exploitation of people. It can also be achieved by workers learning to recognise and be sensitive to processes that are common within agencies such as marginalisation, scapegoating, labelling, victim blaming, denial and inaction.

3   AOP involves workers being open to challenge and change, and to making themselves vulnerable. It means having the security to be able

to admit that it is possible to be wrong, and being prepared to be subject to personal transformation.

4   AOP involves learning to challenge abuses of power, whether intentional or unintentional, covert or overt. For example, it may involve arguing for a service user's rights in a multidisciplinary meeting or case conference. It may involve questioning policies and procedures (and whistle blowing!). It may involve listening seriously to and acting on the criticisms of those who speak from another perspective (black workers, perhaps). It may involve challenging the remarks and actions of colleagues.

5   AOP involves ensuring that the power users should have – their legal rights, the power of knowledge, of participation in decision making, the possibility of appeals and complaints, etc. – is available to them; that is, it is known and accessible, perhaps through the provision of advocates. This means ensuring that people are present when decisions are made which affect their lives or the lives of those close to them. And ensuring that they are prepared, informed and able to participate and know where and how they can seek redress if they do not agree with decisions.

6   AOP involves creating new sources of power where possible, by supporting or initiating self-help or common interest groups; by seeking out resources needed for people to make choices; by developing new policies and procedures which give people greater rights of involvement and participation; and by harnessing the power of new information technologies such as the internet.

7   AOP involves understanding the processes used by people who are or who feel powerless and not blaming them for adopting those responses. These are processes such as passivity, adopting dominant norms, manipulations, staying separate, presenting a 'negative' challenge, accentuating difference, and even uprising and revolt.

8   AOP involves dealing with the personal pain and devaluation often felt by people who are oppressed by offering support, counselling, assertiveness and awareness training to those who have little sense of self-esteem or who have been abused.

9   AOP involves recognising the strengths, insights and survival skills that many oppressed people develop, strengths of self knowledge and understanding. It also involves recognising the strengths in diverse forms of 'family life' or the value of lay approaches to dealing with ill health. And it means being sceptical about the explanations of professionals, academics, politicians and all who occupy positions of authority and power.

10   AOP involves monitoring and evaluating the outcomes of intervention because good intentions are not enough. This can be done by,

for instance, obtaining user feedback, ethnic monitoring, and ongoing training.

Conclusion

The antecedents of contemporary anti-racism are indeed very long and deep rooted. Anti-racist social work began as a social movement born out of black demands for justice and equality. While being wary of the task ahead, much progress has been made. However, it must always be remembered that without political struggle institutions and governments do not change. It was not the Jack Straw of the freshly elected New Labour government that was able to deliver up the Macpherson Report but Stephen Lawrence's parents and the campaign group. Nevertheless, one should not ignore the fact that politics is always a combination of action, passion and ideology. Ultimately, the true value of the theoretical devices of postmodernism and poststructuralism is their application to politics and practice. In the final reckoning, perhaps opposition struggles such as anti-racism are always born out of a critical praxis, and social movements emerge when enough people are prepared to stand up and be counted. This, in my view, will require that workers adopt the 'five Cs':

- *Cause* – what do I stand for and is my practice connected to wider social and political ideals?
- *Commitment* – am I really serious about change?
- *Collaboration* – do I believe that only by working with others I can achieve change?
- *Creativity* – what new ideas, strategies, analyses can I bring?
- *Critical thinking* – am I employing my intellectual faculties to confront inappropriate dominant ideas about humanity and the social world?

References

Chahal, K. and Julienne, L. (1999) *'We Can't All be White!': Racist Victimisation in the UK*, Bristol: Polity/Joseph Rowntree Foundation.

Derrida, J. (1978) *Writing and Difference*, London: Routledge and Kegan Paul.

Frankenberg, R. (1993) *White Women, Race Matters: The Social Construction of Whiteness*, Minneapolis, MN: University of Minnesota Press.

Gilroy, P. (1987) *There Ain't No Black in the Union Jack*, London: Hutchinson.

Hall, S. (1992) 'New Ethnicities', in Donald, J. and Rattansi, A. (eds), *'Race', Culture and Difference*, London: Sage.

Macpherson, W. (1999) *The Stephen Lawrence Enquiry*, London: Stationery Office.

Rattansi, A. (1994) '"Western" Racisms, Ethnicities and Identities in a "Post-Modern" Frame', in Rattansi, A. and Westwood, S., *Racism, Modernity, and Identity on the Western Front*, Cambridge: Polity Press.

Scarman, Lord (1981) *The Brixton Disorders 10–12 April 1981*, London: HMSO.

Sivanandan, A., at www.homebeats.co.uk/resources/lawrence.htm (accessed 10 January 2000).

Solomos, J. (1999) *Race and Racism in Contemporary Britain*, Basingstoke: Macmillan.

Williams, E. (1966) *Capitalism and Slavery*, New York: Capricorn Books.

Chapter 6

Managing diversity and countering discrimination in health services

Rabbi Julia Neuberger and Naaz Coker

Introduction

Drawing on a range of evidence relating to service delivery and employment practices, this chapter addresses the impact of discrimination on the health outcomes and employment opportunities of people from black and minority ethnic groups (BMEs). We indicate why the pursuit of race equality is particularly important in the NHS in the early twenty-first century, invoking the duty of social justice inherent in all public services and highlighting recent policy and legislative initiatives that give impetus to addressing race discrimination. We draw attention to examples of 'good practice' in local NHS equal opportunity policies, and conclude with an assessment of health advocacy as an anti-discriminatory strategy.

Discrimination, health and the NHS

There is a growing body of evidence indicating that people from BME communities carry a higher burden of poor health, premature deaths and long-term chronic ill health than other groups in the population. For example, the incidence of chronic heart disease is nearly 50 per cent higher among Pakistanis and Bangladeshis, taken together, than among whites (Nazroo, 1997: 48), and in Bradford, an unpublished study cited by Kernohan (1998) indicated that the mortality rate from ischaemic heart disease among Asian men of 45–64 is more than twice the rate for non-Asian men in the same age group. Hypertension rates among Black Caribbean women are 80 per cent higher than among white women, with mortality rates also being raised (Nazroo, 1997: 49) The rate of stillbirths to Pakistani women is twice the rate for women as a whole (Henley and Schott, 1996). Refugees and asylum seekers, who are one of the most vulnerable groups, experience multiple deprivation which can have a severe impact on their health. Their experiences make them a high risk group for mental ill health which is compounded by problems of displacement, resettlement, poverty and language difficulties (Karmi, 1998).

These differences are only partly understood but it is clear that they reflect socio-environmental determinants of health more than ethnicity as such. BME groups with the worst general health are also those who live in the most deprived localities and on the lowest incomes (Social Exclusion Unit, 2000). The determinant of income alone, however, does not explain why BME groups are more often ill than white people. The experience of discrimination and racism and its impact on the health of black people is well documented. Racism and particularly institutional racism in the NHS increases inequality and injustice which contribute to anxiety and avoidable ill health (SILKAP, 2000; Karmi, 1998). While there has been much controversy as to whether racism on the part of doctors is a contributory factor or not, high rates of compulsory admission of black people to mental health in-patient facilities, compared with white people, have been consistently documented. Even allowing related factors to be controlled for, such as age, a diagnosis of psychosis and the risk of being violent, black Caribbean patients are still around twice as likely to be compulsorily admitted as white patients (Singh *et al.*, 1998).

From an employment perspective, sadly, discrimination remains a feature of NHS employment practices (NHS Executive, 1999: 3). As a major employer, a provider of services to people at the times of their greatest need and as a national institution influencing wider attitudes to social justice, the NHS has a vital role in embracing diversity in its workforce. Yet despite its foundation on the principle of fairness and its responsibility to serve all sections of the community equally, there is copious evidence in London as elsewhere that health services are falling well short of this aspiration. Black people continue to face disadvantages and discrimination in employment. As Williams (1989: 76) suggests, the health service has relied heavily on black staff to occupy low level positions, such as those in auxiliary nursing, and in the 'domestic' grades for a considerable period. Similarly recruitment to the less desirable branches of medicine, such as general medicine, psychiatry and old age, has also relied on the supply of doctors from the Commonwealth countries. Ward (1993: 172) comments that 'the West Indies were targeted for nurse recruitment, and India and Pakistan, and other former colonies, were called in to provide doctors'.

Recent media attention has focused on the fact that black nurses are leaving the NHS in disproportionate numbers and the number of black women entering the nursing profession is declining significantly. During the last decade the NHS has taken several initiatives to create equality in employment as well as programmes to develop and promote BME staff (NHS Executive, 1996). However discrimination remains a feature of NHS employment practices as demonstrated by the lack of black staff at senior levels in the service. Eight per cent of NHS nursing and midwifery staff are from BME communities, yet under one per cent of nurse executive directors are from BME groups (UKCC, 1999).

Despite the acute shortage of nursing and midwifery staff, the health service is finding it difficult to attract and retain staff from BME communities; for example, only 2.6 per cent of nurses under the age of 25 years are from BME groups, whereas nearly 25 per cent of nurses over 55 years are from these communities. That shortage of young black people taking up nursing as a career has focused attention on the experiences of the first generation of black nurses in the NHS – evidence that the problems they faced have discouraged the present generation of young people from joining the profession (Buchan *et al.*, 1998; Gerrish *et al.*, 1996; UKCC, 1999).

There is also ample evidence of racism in the medical workforce (Ward, 1993), ranging from entry into medical schools to training and support during employment, receipt of merit awards, the number of complaints that are upheld against black doctors. Collard (1995) cites a PSI study in which 66 per cent of black nursing staff stated that they 'had difficulties with patients for ethnic reasons', and 37 per cent of black nursing staff reported that they 'had difficulties with colleagues for ethnic reasons'. So the NHS has to be seriously challenged to become a fair employer of black people.

Demographic profile of minority communities in Britain

Within the last twenty years, the demographic composition of Britain has undergone significant change. To be understood, these changes have to be seen in a historical and socio-economic context. It has long been recognised that in the 1950s and 1960s, migrants from the Caribbean and Indian subcontinent formed a replacement population in towns and cities experiencing an exodus of indigenous inhabitants away from inner cities (Peach 1968). According to Peach:

> both West Indian and Asian immigrant groups formed replacement populations. They were drawn into jobs that were proving unable to attract white workers. These jobs were overwhelmingly urban, and were found mostly in large city centres that were declining in population.
>
> (Peach, 1984: 215–16)

In the UK as a whole, about one person in sixteen is from a minority ethnic group (Office for National Statistics, 2000). In London, that figure is nearer one in four, while in the boroughs of Brent and Newham about half of all residents come from a minority ethnic group (London Research Centre, 1997). The largest minority ethnic groups in Britain are those from South Asia, the Caribbean and Ireland, though the Irish group, since its members are classified as white, is generally identified in many official surveys as belonging to the majority rather than to a minority. There are also significant numbers of Chinese, African and Eastern European people in the UK. An estimated 250,000 refugees live in the UK, about 85 per cent of whom, according to one study cited by SILKAP (2000: 1) reside in Greater London.

However, it is worth emphasising that, especially in London, the terms 'black' and 'minority ethnic' are becoming increasingly difficult to define as people's perceptions of their own identity from ethnicity and social perspectives change (Gilroy, 1987; Tizard and Phoenix, 1993). Around 45 per cent of London's black and minority ethnic labour force were born in this country and many identify themselves as Londoners (London Research Centre, 1997).

Most ethnic minority populations are concentrated in urbanised parts of the country. More than two thirds live within the four connurbations of Greater London, Greater Manchester, West Yorkshire and West Midlands (Social Exclusion Unit, 2000). This distribution of black and ethnic minority populations does not, however, mean that the health of these groups should be the sole concern of the big cities.

Social Exclusion and race inequality

Social Exclusion is the government's preferred term term for describing groups or communities of people who suffer from a combination of linked problems such as unemployment, low skills base, low income, poor housing, high crime environments, poor health and family breakdown or social marginalisation. All these factors lead to social isolation of individuals or groups. Institutional and cultural discrimination and lack of access to public services can further increase social exclusion. Data summarised by the Social Exclusion Unit (2000: para. 2.2) suggests that ethnic minority disadvantage cuts across all aspects of deprivation. Taken as a whole, 'ethnic minority groups are more likely than the rest of the population to live in poor areas, be unemployed, have low incomes, live in poor housing, have poor health and be victims of crime'.

People from some BME groups are excluded due to multiple factors. They are exceptionally concentrated in many of the deprived areas around towns and cities and experience all the problems that affect other people in these areas (Burden and Hamm, 2000: 187). In addition, they experience the consequences of racial discrimination and racial harassment. Services that do not meet their immediate and long-term needs combined with language and cultural barriers and a lack of general information on ways of accessing support services increase this isolation further. People reporting experiences of racially motivated verbal abuse were 50 per cent more likely to report fair or poor health than those who had not experienced racial harassment. People experiencing racially motivated assault or damage to their property were more than twice as likely to report fair or poor health (SILKAP, 2000: 2, citing the Fourth National Survey of Ethnic Minorities).

More than 80 per cent of the Pakestani and Bangladeshi populations live in households that have incomes which are less than half the national average. This compares with figures of 40 per cent for African-Caribbeans, and 34 per cent for Chinese. The statistic for people in England and Wales as a whole who are living in such households is 28 per cent (Berthoud, 1997, cited in Social Exclusion Unit, 2000). The unemployment rate for men from ethnic minorities is twice as high as that for white men, and there is a similar pattern for women, although the rates of unemployment are not quite as high for ethnic minority women as for men. There is a parti-cular concentration of ethnic minority men in the service industries: over 60 per cent of Bangladeshi men work in restaurants, half as cooks or waiters. Indian and Pakistani women are particularly likely to work in manufacturing areas such as textiles, or in retail, while black women are significantly more likely to work in health or social work than white women (Sly *et al.*, 1998: 605–8).

Why is race equality even more relevant now?

The inequalities in the health of the nation (Townsend *et al.*, 1988) have been subject to extensive debate and policy initiatives over a number of years (Department of Health, 1992, 1997, 1998, 2000). Many of the 'problems' and needs have been long identified but are still awaiting resolution. As long ago as 1980, the Black Report on inequalities in health, reported that:

> one of the most important dimensions of inequality in contemporary Britain is race. Immigrants to this country from the so-called New Commonwealth, whose ethnic identity is clearly visible in the colour of their skin are known to experience greater difficulty in finding work and adequate housing. Given these disabilities, it is to be expected that they might also record higher than average rates of mortality.
>
> (Townsend *et al.*, 1988: 50)

The Macpherson Report

The Macpherson Report (1999) has now given a momentum and legitimacy to action against racism rarely seen in the UK before. It created a clear definition of institutional racism that moved away from blaming and label-ling individuals as racist to an understanding that long-standing practices can cause organisations to discriminate unwittingly. This has enabled us to take a new approach to racism, moving away from 'witch-hunting', and attributing racism to particular individuals or groups, towards a search for positive solutions. Institutional racism is defined in the Macpherson Report as:

The collective failure of an organisation to provide an appropriate and professional service to people because of their colour, culture or ethnic origin. It can be seen or detected in processes, attitudes and behaviour which amount to discrimination through unwitting prejudice, ignorance, thoughtlessness and racist stereotyping which disadvantage minority ethnic people.

(Macpherson, 1999: 28)

Although the Macpherson Inquiry focused on the police service, note was taken of Robin Oakley's view that: 'it could be said that institutional racism . . . is in fact pervasive throughout the culture and institutions of the whole of British society, and is in no way specific to the police service' (ibid.: 26). The report stressed the need for every institution to examine its policies and practices, to guard against disadvantaging sections of the community. It suggested that 'a colour-blind approach fails to take account of the nature and needs of the person or people involved'. Treating every one the same will not provide equal opportunities for people who are substantially disadvantaged and discriminated against and whose culture may not be understood.

It can be expected that institutional racism and more widespread societal racism contributes to the process by which black and ethnic minority groups continue to be over-represented among the unemployed, among low income groups, among pupils excluded from school and among those occupying poor housing. All these factors are associated with poorer health.

Overt racism from individuals remains a very significant problem in the UK, as suggested by findings of the Fourth National Survey of Ethnic Minorities cited earlier. Just over one quarter of white respondents had a preference for a doctor of their own 'ethnic origin' and while 60 per cent of this group stated that this was because they had difficulty understanding a non-white doctor, and thus, for them, overt racism cannot be assumed to be proven, for the other 40 per cent the reasons given suggest, 'more clearly contained elements of prejudice' (Nazroo, 1997: 122–3). It has been estimated that there were 382,000 racist incidents in England and Wales during 1995, but only 12,200 of these incidents were reported to and recorded by police (British Crime Survey and Home Office, cited in Social Exclusion Unit, 2000, para. 2.46).

Race relations legislation and racial discrimination

The Race Relations Act 1976 was a turning point in combating racial discrimination in Britain (Runnymede Trust, 1979). Under the Act, it became illegal to discriminate on racial grounds in employment, education and in the provision of services and goods. 'Racial grounds' include colour, race, nationality (including citizenship) or ethnic or national origins. The Act distinguishes two main types of racial discrimination:

- direct discrimination – treating a person, on racial grounds, less favourably than others are or would be in similar circumstances; and
- indirect discrimination – applying a requirement or condition which puts people from a particular racial group at a disadvantage compared to others.

The Race Relations Act does not allow positive discrimination; an employer cannot try to change the balance of the workforce by selecting someone mainly because he or she is from a particular racial background. However, it does allow positive action to prevent discrimination or as redress for past discrimination. This might include providing training for people from a particular racial group, or by encouraging people from that group to apply for certain kinds of work. The aim of positive action is to ensure equality of opportunity. Selection itself must be based on merit and all applicants treated equally.

The Race Relations (Amendment) Act received Royal Assent in November 2000. The amended Act strengthens and extends the scope of the 1976 Act, and is targeted specifically at the public sector – the NHS, schools, the police service, local councils and government offices. Instead of the previous duty simply not to behave in discriminatory ways, all public services now have a positive duty to promote equality in every area of their work (Home Office, 2000).

Anti-racism and equal opportunity

Anti-racism is more than implementing equal opportunity policies (Dominelli, 1988: 136). It requires an understanding and recognition of the processes and expression of racism including the power relationships between black and white people. It seeks to challenge racist assumptions and cultural stereotypes in favour of policies, structures and practices that are sensitive to, and valuing of, cultural differences. Nonetheless, the focus on 'difference' between cultures in anti-racist practice has been criticised for its tendency to homogenise ethnic identities and reify cultural boundaries, as well as to affect, in a similar way identities pertaining to disability and sexuality. In this respect, the efforts in the NHS to link equality with quality, and the increasing emphasis on 'managing diversity' as opposed to managing minority problems, are suggestive of a new organising theme and language for the pursuit of equal opportunities in public services into the twenty-first century. There are of course a number of dimensions to equal opportunity understood in this broader sense. At the political level, equality means providing people with a fair chance in life, in terms of ensuring a so-called level playing field, of opportunities to participate and progress. At the organisational level, in public services, it means not just treating all people as if they were the same, which would simply reproduce existing forms of inequality, but rather developing frameworks for redressing the imbalances society creates between groups of people. In a culturally and ethnically diverse society with pronounced social inequalities, racial discrimination and prejudice, this organisational imperative builds on the duty of ensuring social justice that is implicit in the role of public services. Equal opportunities practice which has a principal focus on redressing imbalances, and which covers both employment of staff and the provision of services, must therefore be the concern of every public service.

Addressing discrimination in service provision

There is clear evidence that BME individuals and groups experience barriers to accessing health care services which may in turn affect their health outcomes. For example, Airey and Evans (1999) reporting a national survey of NHS patients seen in general practice found that:

- Almost half of Asian women reported being unable to see a female GP either always or sometimes (c.f. 25 per cent white women and 35 per cent black Caribbean or African women) (p. 192);
- Seeing a GP of a person's own ethnic group is most important for those who do not speak English (among Chinese people, 17 per cent of English speakers thought it important, compared with 41 per cent of non-English speakers) (p. 193);
- White patients were more likely to say they were seen by their GP soon enough (81 per cent against 63 per cent for ethnic minorities) (p. 106);
- 32 per cent of Bangladeshi and 33 per cent of Chinese patients said GP consultation was too short (c.f. 25 per cent white and 21 per cent black Caribbean) (p. 118); and
- 19 per cent of minority ethnic patients have wanted to complain in the past months but have not done so (c.f. 11 per cent of white patients) (p. 226).

Maxwell and Streetly's (1998) study of sickle-cell sufferers found that many of them were unable to control their pain because they had not been helped and advised to do so by health service workers: many GPs lacked knowledge about sickle-cell disorders and could not advise patients on self-care; patients often felt stigmatised and patronised by health workers (see also Chapple and Anionwu, 1998).

The National Household Survey suggested that BME groups (particularly Pakistanis and Bangladeshis) appear to consult GPs more often than white people. The paradox is that in contrast to their high consulting rates, BME groups make lower than average use of hospital services. The reasons for such differences are not completely understood, but they are not solely accounted for by the reluctance of BME patients to undergo hospital procedures. Nzegwu (1993: 107) found that African and Asian patients reported longer waiting times to see GPs than white patients, even though the place of access was usually in an appointment-run facility, and that satisfaction with GPs was noticeably lower among non-manual African and Asian patients.

Equal access, equal shares and equal treatment

As noted above, *equal access* is not about opening the service doors to all comers, nor is it about using a 'colour blind' approach, offering the same service to everyone and assuming that each person will therefore receive an appropriate service. It means offering flexible, responsive services in which differing needs are identified and accommodated so that each person benefits equally. In other words, needs are addressed in such a way that each 'consumer' will come away with a level of personal satisfaction with what is provided and how it is provided. Henley and Schott go on to add that:

> equal access to services cannot be achieved by ad hoc measures or by individuals working alone. It must be a fundamental policy of the organisation, understood and implemented by everyone responsible for managing and providing care, and backed up by training and practical support.
>
> (Henley and Schott, 1996: 49)

It means that there will be availability of translation services, that people will be accorded respect and dignity and that professionals will use more culturally sensitive approaches.

Equal shares are based on assessment of needs and demands. Services for minority communities have often been provided as ad hoc projects with external funding resulting in 'stop–start' initiatives and considered as added-on services. The critical issue is that services are integrated within the overall health service; in other words they are mainstreamed into core services. *Equal treatment* means different treatments based on the same quality standard.

The problems with NHS initiatives in relation to minority ethnic groups have generally been of three main kinds. First, they are 'patchy' in nature, targeted at catchment areas where there is low take up of services by minority ethnic populations and low levels of interest among them in employment positions within the service (NHS Executive, 1999; Moran and Simpkin, 2000: 98–9). Moreover, there is a paucity of research into variations in access to and use of services by sub groups of BME communities, with the distinctiveness of homogeneous, unchanging cultures continuing to be presented (Rawaf *et al.*, 1998). Second, and related to the 'patchiness' issue, there is still a prevalent belief in a universal and monocultural standard service that will be suitable for all: thus change is often directed at getting minorities into the NHS, rather than changing the NHS (NHS Executive, 1999). In so far as black people continue to be seen, in this way, as presenting problems to be solved rather than as partners to co-create innovative designs for services, the NHS remains a service that 'does things to people' rather than with them. The responsibility for change is one sided. Third, there is no statutory or executive requirement for service providers to analyse the equity of inputs, processes or outcomes in the populations they serve.

In order to improve service access and health outcomes for people from BME communities, health service providers need to:

- understand their population – in terms of numbers, economic status, social background, cultural and religious characteristics, including subcultural characteristics;
- understand their health needs, including their disease patterns and concepts of health;
- listen to communities and involve them in decision making, i.e. seek to achieve participation not just consultation;
- develop long-term staff competence at all levels – ensure understanding of anti-racism and cultural awareness is developed among workers;
- begin to eradicate institutional racism; and
- relate to, and treat the members of diverse communities as whole beings rather than just as containers of health deficits.

Health advocacy

Advocacy involves more than just translation and interpreting; it is also about representing the client's needs and requires a longer-term relationship with the client. Advocacy allows cross-cultural communication which simple language translations do not (for instance, because of different concepts of health and illness). Advocacy for minority ethnic groups works at individual, group and population levels. At the individual level it provides that interpreting for non-English speakers is available, that sources of support are identified, and that help for the interpretation and support is secured from mainstream services. At the group level, it provides for health education, promotion of the use of services (such as, for example, screening and immunisation), and that people's awareness of their rights is increased. At the level of population, health advocacy works by means of encouraging services to provide better support to groups within the population and assisting in the planning of health care or health improvement programmes. Without a strong advocacy voice, and the development of these forms of support, many minority groups get ignored or marginalised by mainstream services (SILKAP, 2000). The training of health workers gives little attention to diversity issues, so the educational role they play is important.

However, health advocacy still faces major problems in gaining acceptance in the mainstream because its benefits are not widely accepted (the evidence base remains weak from lack of research). It is also marginal to most organisations' lists of priorities (the NHS is faced with major tasks like developing Primary Care Groups (PCGs), implementing clinical governance and meeting Government targets, which divert attention away from diversity and equity issues). Advocacy services frequently receive short-term funding, making it hard to develop staff and infrastructure. A King's Fund study of voluntary sector funding from the NHS found that the amounts secured were small and that very little of it was for advocacy work or capacity building (Mocroft et al., 1999).

The King's Fund is, at the time of writing (April, 2001) concentrating on developing health advocacy in London, and key areas of interest are: integration of health advocacy into NHS mainstream services (so as to secure funding and influence); means of developing formal training, regulation and accreditation for health advocacy (so that professionals and other specialists in this area may improve their standing); and ways of helping voluntary sector organisations that are active in this area to get statutory sector contracts (in order to build their capacity).

Addressing inequality in employment

As a major employer (the NHS employs a million people in all areas of the country), the health service can do much to reduce social inequalities by creating equality in recruitment and retention policies and practices. This will benefit patients and the service. As the NHS Executive (1999: 7) notes, the government's inclusiveness goal 'of ensuring that public services meet the needs of all citizens', can only be succesfully achieved by the NHS 'playing its part, as the largest employer in the UK, in national and local partnership action for community renewal, tackling social exclusion and health inequalities'.

How is the NHS doing on equal opportunities?

An NHS Executive (1998) survey of equal opportunities in 420 NHS Trusts found:

- 85 per cent said they had a member of staff responsible for equal opportunities in employment – but most spent under 10 per cent of their time on equal opportunities work;

- 98 per cent of Trusts have an equal opportunities policy – of which 90 per cent related to ethnic minorities, 81 per cent to faith groups, 77 per cent to sexuality and 67 per cent to age;
- 90 per cent of Trusts collect equal opportunities data on recruitment (usually ethnicity, gender and disability). Most trusts keep data on workforce, but few monitor promotions, redundancies, dismissals or training;
- 25 per cent of Trusts said that Board members attached high priority to equal opportunities, 58 per cent said medium, 13 per cent low and two trusts said none.

Drawing on both the examples given in this survey, and on King's Fund programmes, the following instances of good practice in NHS equal employment opportunities can be highlighted.

Barts and the London NHS Trust appointed a Community Communications Officer, within its communications department, to further the process of making links with local people. The Trust has opened a Muslim prayer room in the London Hospital, following on from meetings with the East London Mosque and with other community groups. The London Trust has also made provision for more single-sex wards and instituted separate mortuary arrangements to meet the requirements of Muslim and Jewish funerals. There is a quarterly newsletter for community groups and the Trust works with them on local events, including events where people can comment on hospital services and to find out about career opportunities.

Blackburn, Hyndburn and Ribble Valley Health Care NHS Trust has aimed to overcome poor representation of ethnic minorities in training for nursing and professions allied to medicine, and poor retention of minorities by: (a) setting up cultural awareness sessions and fair selection training for managers (ensuring that every selection panel has at least one person who has undergone training); (b) setting targets for ethnic minority representation in the workforce; and (c) monitoring recruitment patterns so as to identify problem areas. The Trust has also introduced a policy on flexible working including a pilot project of flexible shifts for nurses working on annualised hours.

Bradford Hospitals NHS Trust has pursued a strategy for equal opportunities through a high-level steering group, to which a full-time post is dedicated. Action taken has included: training on equal opportunities and discrimination in relation to recruitment and selection; the promotion of job advertisements in ethnic minority publications; and the provision of specialist courses for career development linked to improved use of appraisals. Every new member of staff attends cultural awareness training, and senior staff attend regular briefings on equal opportunities. The Trust has also compiled a comprehensive database of workforce data, which is used to produce an annual report for the Board.

Newham Community Health Service NHS Trust has provided for leadership of equality issues to be given by a non-executive director on the Trust Board. At staff level, leadership is by means of a Health and Race Action Group comprising both senior managers and members of community groups. Three staff members have been appointed to the BEL Programme at the King's Fund, a programme which offers positive action training for black staff with leadership potential, one of whom rewrote the Trust's equal opportunities policy as part of her course. There is a training guarantee that a minimum of three days a year are devoted to minority ethnic issues and there is a focus on initiatives that tackle both staff and community needs.

Nottingham Community Health NHS Trust has developed an equal opportunities project to cover all aspects of the issue. A key part of its innovative policy on harassment is aimed at shifting the burden of proof from the victim to the perpetrator, while the victim has recourse to two support workers (one black, one Asian) who are appointed via a ballot of minority ethnic staff. The two workers are given time away from normal duties to provide support outside usual line management structures. There is mandatory race awareness training for all staff and the Trust monitors recruitment and progression through the workforce, including pay and full/part-time status, by means of reviews undertaken by an equal opportunities monitoring group.

Redbridge NHS Trust has worked with the King's Fund to encourage Asian women to seek the help of mental health services (having identified their significant under-use of such services) through the production of information leaflets in Asian languages and networking in existing community women's groups.

Conclusion

There is a political impetus for action against racism – ministers have promised tough action to tackle violence and harassment against NHS workers, particularly where it is racially motivated. Health inequalities are a policy priority. Health Improvement Programmes give health organisations an unprecedented opportunity to work with partners outside the NHS to tackle the causes of ill health and to work with minority ethnic communities to find workable solutions to the health problems they face.

Service provision and employment opportunities are two sides of the same coin and neither can be tackled in isolation. Both require similar action, which should be pursued with equal vigour.

In service provision, it means looking at what services are provided and the degree to which they meet the needs of all the different communities served. Specific services may need to be developed for communities with particular needs, or changes made to the way mainstream services are provided in order to reach out to groups who cannot access them, do not use them or do not benefit from them. The use of health services and treatments is influenced by people's health beliefs, which in turn are shaped by cultural influences. Although some health beliefs may be at odds with those held by health professionals, within every culture there are norms and values which promote good health. Health professionals need to learn to work with the positive aspects of different cultures and not just focus on the cultural barriers.

In employment, action means examining institutional practices such as employment, promotion, reward systems, training and development practices. These should be monitored for inadvertent bias, racial discrimination and harassment, and in order to find ways of eradicating them. A tougher line must be taken on those who abuse staff or patients.

References

Airey, C. and Erens, B. (eds) (1999) *National Surveys of NHS Patients: General Practice, 1998*, a survey for the NHS Executive, London: Stationery Office.

Bhugra, D. and Bahl, V. (1999) *Ethnicity: An Agenda for Mental Health*, London: Policy Studies Institute.

Buchan, J., Seccombe, J. and Smith, G. (1998) *Nurses Work: An Analysis of the UK Nursing Labour Market*, Aldershot: Ashgate.

Burden, T. and Hamm, T. (2000) 'Responding to socially excluded groups', in Percy-Smith, J. (ed.) *Policy Responses to Social Exclusion: Towards Inclusion?*, Buckingham: Open University Press.

Chapple, J. and Anionwu, E.N. (1998) 'Genetic Services', in Rawaf, S. and Baal, V. (eds) *Assessing Health Needs of People from Minority Ethnic Groups*, London: Royal College of Physicians.

Collard, A. (1995) 'Training in racial harassment issues for community staff', *Nursing Times*, vol. 91, no. 32.

Department of Health (1992) *The Health of the Nation: A Strategy for Health in England*, London: HMSO.

Department of Health (1997) *The New NHS: Modern, Dependable*, London: Stationery Office.

Department of Health (2000) *The NHS Plan: A Plan for Investment, A Plan for Reform*, London: Stationery Office.

Dreyer, F. and Whitehead, M. (1997) *Health Inequalities*, London: Stationery Office.

Department of Health (1998) *Our Healthier Nation: A Contract for Health*, London: Stationery Office.

Dominelli, L. (1988) *Anti-Racist Social Work: A Challenge for White Practitioners and Educators*, Basingstoke: Macmillan.

Gerrish, K. Husband, C. and McKenzie, J. (1996) *Nursing for a Multi-ethnic Society*, Buckingham: Open University Press.

Gilroy, P. (1987) *There Ain't No Black in the Union Jack*, London: Hutchinson.

Henley, A. and Schott, J. (1996) *Culture, Religion and Childbearing in a Multi-racial Society*, Oxford: Butterworth–Heinemann.

Home Office (2000) Race Relations (Amendment) Act, London: Stationery Office.

Johnson, M.R.D. (1987) 'Towards racial equality in health and welfare: what progress?', *New Community*, vol. X1V, no. 2

Karmi, G. (1998) 'Refugees', in Rawaf, S. and Baal, V. (eds) *Assessing Health Needs of People from Minority Ethnic Groups*, London: Royal College of Physicians.

Kernohan, E.E.M. (1998) 'Heart health', in Rawaf, S. and Baal, V. (eds), op. cit.

King's Fund (1998) *National Survey of NHS Patients (General Practice)*, London: King's Fund.

London Research Centre (1997) *Cosmopolitan London: Past, Present and Future*, London: London Research Centre.

Maxwell, K. and Streetly, A. (1998) *Living with Sickle Cell Pain*, London: Guy's, King's and St Thomas' School of Medicine.

MacPherson, D. (1999) *The Stephen Lawrence Inquiry*, London: Stationery Office.

McNaught, A. (1987) *Health Action and Ethnic Minorities*, London: Bedford Square Press.

Mocroft, I., Pharaoh, C. and Romney-Alexander, D. (1999) *Healthy Relationships*, West Malling, Kent: Charities Aid Foundation.

Moran, G. and Simpkin, M. (2000) 'Social exclusion and health', in Percy-Smith, J. (ed.) *Policy Responses to Social Exclusion: Towards Inclusion?*, Buckingham: Open University Press.

NHS Executive (1996) *Annual Report – 1995/96*, London: HMSO.

NHS Executive (1998) *Equal Opportunities and Monitoring in NHS Trusts: A Survey of 420 NHS Trusts in England and 25 Case Studies of Good Practice in Equal Opportunities*, London: Stationery Office.

NHS Executive (1999) *Tackling Racial Harassment in the NHS: A Plan for Action*, London: Stationery Office.

Nazroo, J.Y. (1997) *The Health of Britain's Ethnic Minorities: Findings from a National Survey*, London: Policy Studies Institute.

Nzegwu, F. (1993) *Black People and Health Care in Contemporary Britain*, Reading: International Institute for Black Research.

Office for National Statistics (ONS) (2000) *Social Trends: 30*, London: Stationery Office.

Peach, C. (1968) *Black Migration to Britain: A Social Geography*, London: Oxford University Press.

Peach, C. (1984) 'The force of West Indian island identity in Britain', in Clark, C., Ley, D. and Peach, C. *Geography and Ethnic Pluralism*, London: Allen and Unwin.

Percy-Smith, J. (ed.) (2000) *Policy Responses to Social Exclusion: Towards Inclusion?*, Buckingham: Open University Press.

Rawaf, S., Owen, F. and Gilffilian, V. (1998) in Rawaf, S. and Baal, V. (eds) op. cit.

Runnymede Trust (1979) *A Review of the Race Relations Act 1976*, London: Runnymede Trust.

Social Exclusion Unit (2000) *Preventing Social Exclusion*, London: Stationery Office.

SILKAP (2000) *Mapping the Provision of Health Advocacy Services for Black and Minority Ethnic Communities in London*, London: King's Fund.

Singh, S., Croudace, T., Beck, A. and Harrison, G. (1998) 'Perceived ethnicity and the risk of compulsory admission', *Social Psychiatry and Psychiatric Epidemiology*, 33.

Sly, F., Thair, T. and Risdon, A. (1998) 'Labour market participation of ethnic groups', *Labour Market Trends*, vol. 106, no. 12, London: Stationery Office.

Tizard, B. and Phoenix, A. (1993) *Black, White, or Mixed Race? Race and Racism in the Lives of Young People of Mixed Parentage*, London: Routledge.

Townsend, P., Davidson, N. and Whitehead, M. (eds) (1988) *Inequalities in Health: The Black Report and the Health Divide*, Penguin: Harmondsworth.

United Kingdom Central Council for Nursing, Midwifery and Health Visiting (UKCC) (1999) *Fitness for Practice: the UKCC Commission for Nursing and Midwifery Education*, London: UKCC.

Ward, L. (1993) 'Race, equality and employment in the National Health Service', in Ahmad, W.I.U. (ed.) *Race and Health in Contemporary Britain*, Buckingham: Open University Press.

Williams, F. (1989) *Social Policy: A Critical Introduction*, Cambridge: Polity Press.

Chapter 7

Frameworks for anti-discriminatory strategies in the health service

Uduak Archibong

Introduction

There is a long-standing and well-documented pattern of health inequalities in Britain, evident in both health care outcomes and in utilisation of health services, while the gap between health needs and the provision of health services to meet them continues to widen (Baxter, 1997; Department of Health, 2000b). Inequalities in health particularly affect minority ethnic groups because of, among other reasons, disproportionate poverty, discrimination and failure of health service organisations to provide culturally competent care (Ahmad, 1993; Baxter, 1997; Department of Health, 1998a). Lack of competence in handling the needs of culturally diverse users of the health service is a factor in outcomes such as misdiagnosis and inappropriate treatment of Black and Asian people in mental health institutions (Department of Health, 1998d) and in low service utilisation rates among Black and Asian women such as those in uptake of breast and cervical screening. It is also frequently reflected in services providing inappropriate dietary advice and support, inattention to religious requirements, poor interpreting arrangements (Kai, 1999), and poor screening and genetic counselling provisions for sickle cell and thalassaemia (Anionwu, 1996; Department of Health, 1993).

This chapter aims to discuss cultural considerations in health care delivery in relation to countering discrimination in health service. It will describe concepts related to culturally appropriate health care; discuss problems faced in securing a diverse health workforce; consider ways to improve recruitment and retention of people from under-represented groups in the health professions; analyse the role of education and training in promoting culturally competent health care; and identify and discuss approaches to making the NHS a culturally competent organisation. The chapter will not presume to generate a new body of practice strategies and procedures. Rather, it will present a composite of practices and procedures already identified in health care literature and will suggest how they might be adapted to the contemporary NHS environment.

Cultural considerations are as important a component of health and health care for majority as for minority populations, and it should be recognised that culture goes beyond racial, ethnic and linguistic differences (Andrews and Boyle, 1999; Castillo, 1996). Although there are multiple definitions of culture, in essence culture may be considered as an 'invisible blueprint for living' (Jones, 1999), the essence of one's being. The rich array of such blueprints in the UK presents a considerable challenge to service providers. In a variety of health care settings throughout the UK, health care practitioners are increasingly giving care within less visibly distinct cultural contexts to diverse populations including, for example, British-born African women who have been ritually circumcised, English-speaking Eritrean Muslim refugees, and orthodox Jewish families with special needs. The health service will continue to provide care to a pluralistic and multicultural society as refugees, immigrants, diplomatic and military personnel and their dependents move around the world (Callister, 2001). Callister argues that the movement of people around the world creates a 'global village'. As Freedman (2000) suggests, it is in the nature of globalisation that there is virtually no culture in the world that is unaffected by others in reiterating the reality of diversity.

The White Paper, 'The New NHS: Modern, Dependable' (Department of Health, 1997) promises to modernise the health service utilising an approach that combines efficiency and quality with a belief in fairness and partnership. This suggests an approach which both recognises the specific health needs of different groups and is non-discriminatory, individualistic and based on respect for each person's social, intellectual, psychological and cultural needs.

As the health service strives to achieve this goal, there is need for ongoing education, capacity and skill building that will enable health service managers, policy makers and health care providers to effectively utilise cultural competence as a key tool. Recent health policies (Department of Health, 1997, 1998a, 2000b) have explicitly integrated equality objectives into strategic health planning, commissioning of health services and service delivery. In the light of these policy shifts, workforce planning to meet the objectives must clearly take cognisance of the cultural skills and cultural competencies required for health care delivery, with the equality ethos producing the impetus for such an agenda. The present government's drive toward 'improving the quality of care and making services more sensitive to individual needs' thus produces quite specific requirements for the health workforce of the future (Department of Health, 2000a).

Conceptualising culturally appropriate health care

The NHS has a statutory obligation to provide a fair and equitable service shaped around the convenience of patients and clients. In a multicultural society such fairness has the implication that services must be delivered in what has been termed a 'culturally safe' environment by people who are also technically proficient. The principle of cultural competence applies at all levels – organisational, professional and personal. A culturally safe environment is one which promotes care that is non-threatening to individual's cultural identity. However, culture is a dynamic concept which can change rapidly, and those 'elements which have particular significance in defining collective identities are not a permanent expression of some sort of historically determined essence' (Gerrish *et al.*, 1996). In the light of the non-static nature of cultural identity the health professional needs to constantly learn from people about their values, beliefs and practices with a focus on human caring, health and well being (Leininger, 1995).

Cultural appropriateness in health care has been conceptualised in a number of different ways including those of cultural safety, as already mentioned, transcultural communicative competence and cultural competence. The concept of cultural safety reminds health care professionals of their role as custodians of 'personal and corporate culture, attitudes, preconceptions and power' (Nursing Council of New Zealand, 1996). It has a major influence in the training of nurses and midwives in New Zealand, the government of which requires that the future nursing and midwifery workforce be both clinically and culturally safe to practise.

The Nursing Council of New Zealand (1996: 27) defines cultural safety as an outcome of nursing and midwifery education 'that acknowledges power relationships, is regardful of diverse realities and empowers the users of nursing and midwifery services to achieve desired health gains'. The key emphasis of cultural safety is the recognition of how the professional's power and the historical and social factors that surround that power may affect care (McGee, 2000). To be able to provide culturally safe care, professionals are required to work to predetermined standards which are aimed at enabling health care practitioners to reflect on their personal values and attitudes in relation to each individual they meet, and to be open minded and flexible in their approach to people who differ from themselves (Papps and Ramsden, 1996).

Transcultural communicative competence is described by Gerrish *et al.* (1996) as a form of competence requiring that the individual comes to understand the cultural values, behavioural patterns and the rules that underpin interaction in specific cultures. At one level it involves the health professional developing an understanding of the cultural specificity of their own behaviour and ways to modify it to put others at ease. At the same time, it is also important, at this level, for the health professional to understand his or her own cultural values in order to be responsive to others' beliefs and cultures in the context of their work/skills. At another level, transcultural communicative competence aims to enable the health care worker to understand the values and cultural practices which may impinge upon clients' conception of health and illness and of help-seeking behaviour. To be culturally communicative competent the professional needs to have an understanding of communication styles appropriate in diverse cultures.

Cultural competence is a concept which is widely used in the USA and is currently being developed by the National Center for Cultural Competence (Goode and Harrisone, 2000). Cultural competence means 'a dynamic process of framing assumptions, knowledge, and meanings from a culture different than our own' and 'a way of becoming self-aware and of understanding how meaning is assigned' (Bartol and Richardson, 1998). It is a process of working effectively within the cultural context of an individual or community (Campinha-Bacote, 1994b). Campinha-Bacote emphasises the process of becoming culturally competent rather than being culturally competent. Thorpe and Baker (1995) suggest that cultural competence involves a person from one culture being able to think and behave in ways that enable their effective working with members of another culture. This implies a process of continuing development, which enables the practitioner to accept and understand a variety of customs, values and beliefs (Wells, 1995).

Campinha-Bacote (1988, 1994a, 1994b) has developed a model of cultural competence, which includes and builds upon the work of others in the field. Her extensive experience of working as an Advanced Practitioner in Psychiatric Nursing and as a Certified Transcultural Care Nurse have informed this model. The model suggests that cultural competence consists of four elements: cultural awareness, cultural knowledge, cultural skill and cultural encounter. Cultural awareness is developed by, on the one hand, examination of one's own cultural values and culture-specific ways of relating to others, and on the other hand by recognising and developing a sensitivity to the diverse forms of interaction which characterise other cultures. Cultural knowledge is acquired by study of world views and of health beliefs within diverse cultures. Cultural skill is developed by the application of this knowledge to the care-giving process in general terms. Cultural encounter is enabled by means of engaging in cross-cultural care and developing culturally relevant care interventions.

Lipson and Steiger (1996) suggest that, in order to become culturally competent it is essential for the health care worker to develop a cultural perspective consisting of three elements – the self, the other and the context. In respect of the self, the approach requires the professional to examine personal values, beliefs, culture and other factors, which may impinge directly or indirectly on cross-cultural communication. In relation to the 'other', the health care practitioner needs to learn how the values, culture and beliefs of others affect their health, illness and self-care. The final element, context, refers to the circumstances under which the care is given.

Lipson and Steiger go on to advocate three strategies for effective cross-cultural communication – affective, cognitive and behavioural. The affective strategy is based on a non-judgemental, comfortable attitude toward other cultures, recognising that there are many differing culture-bound world views of health and health behaviours which should not only be accepted but also learned from. The cognitive strategy is based on knowledge about other cultures enabling the practitioner to interpret nuances of meaning and relate culture to interpersonal problems. Gaining and applying knowledge about socio-political aspects and about majority–minority cultural relations is an important part of this strategy. The behavioural strategy is based on careful and clear communication, nurturing others to express themselves fully, and being able to recognise and address misunderstandings.

The acquisition of cultural competence at the organisational and individual levels is an ongoing developmental process, rather than one which has a definite endpoint. The process is characterised by movement along the stages of what has been defined as the 'cultural competence continuum' (Cross et al., 1989). Goode and Harrisone (2000) have adapted and expanded the work of Cross et al. to identify six stages in the cultural competence continuum, from cultural destructiveness to cultural proficiency, with the intermediary stages defined as cultural incapacity, cultural blindness, cultural pre-competence and cultural competence. The achievement of cultural proficiency depends on a continuing advancement of the knowledge base of a culturally and linguistically competent practice by means of both research and the development of new forms of treatments, interventions and approaches for health care (Goode and Harrisone, 2000). However there is increasingly a realisation that coherent theories and a research base to guide health care that is culturally competent is yet to be developed (Clinton, 1996; Bartol and Richardson, 1998; Lester, 1998; Meleis, 1996; Smith, 1998). For example, some instruments (i.e. research instruments or procedures for data collection) have been used to measure menopausal symptoms without careful attention to their cultural relevance to those whose symptoms are being measured (Im et al., 1999). There is a need for more research focusing on differentiating the beliefs of women who consistently have regular Pap smears from those who do not (Jennings-Dozier, 1999). Cultural proficiency involves balancing respect for cultural beliefs and practices while maintaining professional standards of care.

Cultural proficiency further entails developing the ability to enhance communication skills in ways that transcend language, as illustrated in the following example by Callister.

A midwife was assigned to a Chinese woman who spoke no English. The client's husband spoke little English, and from his perspective birthing was a woman's work. When the midwife came on her shift, the fearful woman was experiencing the intensity of transition. The physician was present, frustrated by an inability to communicate with the couple, and the midwife could feel the tension that filled the room. The midwife could not speak Chinese either, but she tried to convey a sense of caring, touching the woman, speaking softly, modelling supportive behaviour for her husband, and helping her to relax as much as possible. The atmosphere in the room changed considerably with the calm competence and quiet demeanour of the midwife. Following the birth of a handsome son, the father thanked the midwife and conveyed to her how grateful he was that she spoke Chinese. The midwife tactfully said, 'Thank you, but I don't speak Chinese.' He looked at her in amazement and said with conviction, 'You spoke Chinese to her.'

(Callister, 2001: 212)

This story confirms the importance of transcending purely verbal communication. The midwife showed sufficient acknowledgement of, and concern with, non-verbal cultural cues, including such aspects as voice timbre, touch technique, and gesture to make a difference to the quality of the birth experience of this family.

Securing a diverse health workforce

One of the stated aims of the NHS equality framework (Department of Health, 2000a) is the recruitment, development and retention of a workforce able to provide 'fair, accessible, and appropriate services' which are both of high quality and responsive to the diverse needs of different social groups and individuals. Rashid's (1990) work suggests that the first step to making services accessible to different communities in this way is to achieve a workforce that better reflects the lives of different sections of society. This implies the ability of the health service and educational institutions to recruit and retain members of all sections of the community.

In a joint statement, the Committee of University Vice-Chancellors and Principals and the NHS Executive emphasise the partnership role of the NHS and higher education institutions in:

- developing awareness of what careers in the NHS can offer to the whole of the community;

- nurturing the skills of the potential workforce
- providing new pathways to widen participation.

(Department of Health, 2000b: 14)

The new pathways to widening participation should recognise language differences, differences in religion, employment status, class, culture, differences in abilities and others. Recruitment interventions should not ignore these differences but respond positively to diversity to ensure a representative workforce. Increased representation of disadvantaged groups in the health workforce, particularly at higher levels, is a goal that involves addressing wider social processes, starting with gatekeeping at the recruitment stage (Hastings-Asatourian, 2000). Unstated preferences among white recruiters in favour of white applicants, both reflecting and extending discrimination, like the kinds of social preference expressed outside health settings, have been recognised to be factors in gatekeeping on equality of opportunity. These have to be countered by the NHS's equal opportunities code of practice, which recommends the establishment of consistent criteria for selection to avoid subjectivity and consequent unlawful discrimination (NHS Management Executive, 1994).

The NHS has failed to attract ethnic minority groups into the professions (UKCC, 1999). There is a shortage of young black people taking up nursing as a career as the experiences of the first generation of black nurses in the NHS has deterred young people from joining the profession (University of Central England [UCE], 2001). In 1996–7 only 3.8 per cent of entrants to diploma and degree level pre-registration nursing programmes in England and Wales were black (Buchan et al., 1998). The barriers to recruiting people from diverse backgrounds into the health service have been the subject of both theoretical and research literature (Bharj, 1995; Baxter, 1997; Darr, 1998; UCE, 2001).

Some of the factors which adversely affect attempts to recruit an ethnically diverse health workforce are: racism (Torkington, 1987; Cole, 1987; Pearson, 1987; Platzer, 1988; Baxter, 1988; Lee-Cunin, 1989; ENB, 1998); violation of socio-cultural norms governing the behaviour of women in health work (French et al., 1994); the requirement to provide care to members of the opposite sex to one's own; the requirement to wear a culturally unacceptable uniform in the case of some professional groups (Mares et al., 1985); the low status of some health professions such as nursing (Crowe, 1996; Darr, 1998); the unattractiveness of the prospect of working in a hospital or health-related environment (Darr, 1998); and the lack of role models from minority ethnic groups (Bharj, 1995).

There is also evidence of discriminatory practices in respect of recruitment into medical education. Esmail and Everington (1993) concluded that non-Europeans were less likely to be accepted into medical school. Gatekeeping practices in the recruitment and selection processes for non-medical education have also been highlighted (UCE, 2001; Hastings-Asatourian, 2000). A good example of gatekeeping in nursing is the way in which, historically, black people were directed to undertake the enrolled nurse training route (a lower academic level of nurse training) even though the entrance requirements for the higher level registered nurse training might be fully met (Hicks, 1982a, 1982b; Gerrish *et al.*, 1996). Doyal *et al.*'s (1980) study estimated that nearly one third of enrolled nurses are black, compared with one tenth of registered nurses. Members of disadvantaged groups are still under-represented in key posts in the NHS. They are clustered in the lower grades of nursing and other professional groups within the NHS. Some recruitment materials continue to promote stereotypes and may serve to deter people of under-represented groups from applying for places in health care training programmes.

Navidi sums up concerns regarding racism experienced by minority ethnic people in the health service:

> Racial discrimination operates at all levels in the NHS, right from the processing of application forms through to the top jobs. It presents a concrete ceiling, which keeps talented and qualified ethnic minority staff from the positions they could be filling. Racism operates also on other levels, be it racial harassment or abuse from patients, or unequal disciplinary measures applied to ethnic minority staff.
>
> (Cited in Department of Health, 1997: 3)

There is a dearth of literature on the extent of racial harassment in the NHS. However, available evidence is alarming. As noted by Neuberger and Coker in Chapter 6 of this volume (pp. 82–97), significant minorities of Black and Asian nursing staff indicated in Collard's (1995) study that they have difficulties with colleagues for ethnic reasons while a majority both of Black staff (66 per cent) and Asian staff (58 per cent) reported difficulties with patients for ethnic reasons.

It can be suggested that the main obstacle to recruitment and retention of staff from minority ethnic communities in the health service has been the institutional racism that spreads through both the health service itself and the educational institutions, which provide health care education (Baxter, 1988; Lee-Cunin, 1989; Bharj, 1995). The CRE, in their 1995 annual report, mentioned that concern about racial equality in employment in the health sector has remained high and a number of industrial tribunals have confirmed discriminatory practices. Racism has led to a lack of black role models working in the higher reaches of the service, whose example can be aspired to, long-term problems with work and personal relationships, and low self-esteem and confidence. These problems can be argued to have had a very significant impact on the health workforce.

As part of the wider context of changes and improvements set out in the 1997 White paper on the 'New NHS', the government confirmed its commitment to tackling racism in stating that 'The NHS executive has already asked the NHS Trusts to tackle a range of immediate human resources priorities'. These included measures 'to . . . recognise and deal with racism' (Department of Health, 1997). In view of the disturbing statistics regarding the experience of racism by members of minority groups in the NHS, there is need for early detection of the problems through regular monitoring and evaluation of the outcomes of the NHS's equal opportunities policies. However, as Neuberger and Coker also point out, it is disconcerting to find from the NHS Executive's survey of 420 NHS Trusts in England that none of the specific tasks necessary to evaluate the outcomes of their equal opportunities policies were widely undertaken (Department of Health, 1998b). The survey reports that only a quarter of Trusts stated that their Board attached high priority to equal opportunity issues. With just over a third of Trusts monitoring recruitment and retention against numerical goals, and less than a third assessing employees' views on the policies by survey, the findings raise questions about how Trusts are able to measure their progress in terms of equal opportunities targets.

Nonetheless, there are some indications of a more favourable social environment. In commenting on this social context, the Department of Health notes that the 'Let's Kick Racism out of Football' initiative has considerably lessened the incidence of racist abuse; that increased awareness of landlords and of the police has reduced racial attacks and racial tensions in housing; and that some employers, such as banks and local authorities, have adopted clear and effective policies and procedures for dealing with racial harassment. One NHS Trust, seeking to recruit and retain more staff from minority ethnic groups, saw, over a two-year period, first an upward trend in reported racial harassment from 16 per cent to 42 per cent owing to improved confidence among staff in being able to report incidents, and then a downward trend, to 23 per cent, as the Trust's procedures began to take effect (Department of Health, 1998c).

These examples illustrate that sustained and planned action for intervention is the key to success in continuing to change social attitudes towards discriminatory practices. A policy and legislative framework for such action is provided by the Race Relations Act 1976 and the Race Relations (Amendment) Act (Home Office, 2000). This is a framework within which there is good support for radical approaches to redressing inequalities, and these are the forms of approach which must be adopted if members of disadvantaged groups are to be enabled to enter and stay in the health service in significant numbers.

Promoting culturally competent healthcare education and training

The first NHS equality framework, *The Vital Connection*, highlights the role of health care education in promoting a culturally competent health care (Department of Health, 2000b). The framework emphasises the partnership role in building a diverse workforce that matches up to the challenges of providing equitable and accessible services responsive to differing community needs free of stereotyping and discrimination. The aim is that NHS organisations, educational institutions, professional bodies and other partners develop education and training in such a way as to open up opportunities in the health service to the whole of the community.

Securing a diverse and representative workforce is not sufficient on its own to produce an equitable health service. In order to meet the standards set out in the New National Service Frameworks, the whole workforce needs to be 'educated and developed to appreciate the lives and needs of different groups and communities, and to be able to challenge stereotyping and discrimination' (Department of Health, 2000a).

The key aim of educational preparation of health care professionals is to equip students with the skills and knowledge required for competent, safe and effective practice which is responsive to the varied physical, psychological, social and cultural needs of the individual (Department of Health, 2000a). Students are required to demonstrate their ability to apply technical skills and academic knowledge to clinical practice competently and safely. However the structural dimension of some health care programmes may not always allow for effective preparation of the student in achieving curricula intentions. In a study to evaluate pre-registration undergraduate degrees in Nursing and Midwifery, the ENB (1996) reported that 'curriculum documents express ambitious programme aims . . . some programmes are more appropriately organised than others to achieve these aims'. With particular reference to meeting curricula aims in relation to cultural studies, Gerrish *et al.* (1996) suggest that a number of issues require to be addressed in relation to the adequacy of the preparation of nurses. These include:

- concern with relation to how far lecturers are competent to teach cultural issues;
- difficulties with delivery by external experts in that such input may not support a coherent curriculum;
- problems around the tokenistic practice of bringing in professionals or users from minority ethnic communities to teach elements of the programme where their community's existence is otherwise not acknowledged in the core curriculum;
- lack of involvement of minority ethnic communities in developmental stages of the curriculum;

- scanty coverage of major aspects of culture in curricula, particularly in respect of the socio-political context of the way in which 'ethnic minorities' experience health; and
- lack of institutional support for staff development in the area.

The picture may not be different for other health care education programmes. Although some medical curricula make reference to culture (American Association of Medical Colleges 1984; British Medical Association, 1995), few undergraduate and even fewer postgraduate medical education programmes appear to have any comprehensive coverage of 'multicultural health care' issues (Gill and Green, 1996; Poulton *et al.*, 1986) or to address topics such as prejudice or racism. If the objective of cultural communicative competence is one which is agreed upon, then it follows that health care curricula must explicitly cover areas of cultural awareness, communication and interpersonal skills, valuing and managing diversity, and of working with interpreters and advocates (Kai, 1999). These areas could be taught both as 'stand-alone' topics and as topics which are integrated with other aspects of the curriculum delivered by competent educators. Interactive methods of teaching, such as case studies, group work, simulation, video sessions, and role-play are clearly preferable as teaching methods since didactic approaches, by definition, exclude much of the potential for cross-cultural learning.

Effective communication is central in promoting linguistic competence and in delivering an effective non-discriminatory service. This includes appropriate interpretation services for patients for whom there are language barriers, sign language interpreters for deaf service users and improved written communication. There needs to be a wider strategy to ensure that the health care workforce can communicate effectively with all its users and carers. Pre-registration programmes should be designed to prepare the health professional to perform this role. In addition, NHS organisations and providers of education are to establish good practice standards and models, both as a framework to structure training, accreditation and career routes for interpreters, support and outreach workers, and as a means of training and developing staff to be more effective in engaging those who are not using services because of communication barriers (Department of Health, 2000). Partnership between health authorities, primary care trusts, local authorities, the voluntary sector, NHS Direct and others is key in developing and maintaining appropriate and targeted linguistic competence.

Making the NHS a culturally competent organisation

The NHS as a culture should have culturally defined modes of care delivery and all professionals' practices need to be more culturally appropriate to be effective (Burford, 1997). The role of the health service in nurturing and cherishing its employees and responding to the needs of its distinctive work-force has come under close scrutiny for years. The discrimination that has plagued the NHS over time is well documented (Ahmad, 1993; Gerrish *et al.*, 1996). The government has recognised that the time has come for the NHS, as a large multicultural employer to demonstrate the commitment to the spirit of fairness and equity that underpinned its founding principles (Ahmad and Atkin, 1996) and to promoting the attainment of, and respect for, human rights. Proposed actions to overcome discrimination, in pursuit of these objectives for those employed in the NHS, are identified in *The Vital Connection* (Department of Health, 2000b) as follows:

- modernisation of equal opportunities policies and their integration into the strategic objectives of the NHS;
- taking action to ensure a harassment-free NHS;
- partnership between NHS employers, education consortia and training providers to take positive action to ensure progress for all;
- provision of flexible working and training patterns throughout NHS and educational institutions to enable staff to achieve the balance they need between work and home.

Central to the provision of culturally appropriate care is valuing and working with the existing social networks – including families, informal organisations, and self-help groups – through which individuals find validation in the set-ting of local neighbourhoods. There are wide-ranging health coalitions, which have historically functioned to give voice to the health concerns of minority ethnic communities, and mobilisation around common interests has led to major victories (Braithwaite *et al.*, 2000). Some of these support systems have developed out of resentment by members of minority ethnic communities at the quality of services received within particular health sectors. For example there have been noticeable campaigns by such groups as the African Caribbean Mental Health Association to change the nature of the provision of mental health services to Black and Asian communities, which they deemed to be ethnically insensitive and culturally inappropriate (Fernando, 1991; Sashidharan and Francis, 1993; Woodley Team Support, 1995).

Flexibility, adaptability and the ability of the mainstream health service purchasers to learn from the experiences of the voluntary sector and coalitions in minority ethnic communities are now integral elements in addressing the government modernisation agenda. In addition, the political cues have been given for the health service to participate in the creation and sustenance of extensive and independent minority ethnic community health initiatives, which can work locally and directly with particular communities and give some credence to the idea of 'our healthier nation' (Department of Health, 1998a).

The theme of making the NHS a better place to work has been regularly reiterated, too, in the last few years. If this objective is to be achieved then one of the key challenges to the service in working towards being a culturally competent organisation is that of the formalising of context, structures and procedures in such a way as to promote the building of knowledge. If used appropriately 'organisational knowledge assists in building new competencies and leveraging existing ones' (Stenhouse and Pemberton, 1999). Such knowledge results from both personal and organisational learning and experiences. Each is dependent on the other and linked by organisational context.

The way in which the role of individuals is responded to in NHS culture is crucial to the development of the culturally competent organisation. A staff development programme based on 'valuing and managing diversity' can be seen to be essential to the fostering of appropriate cross-cultural working by all who work in the organisation. Such a training programme could offer participants an opportunity to clarify their personal values, cultural reference points and beliefs and would serve to encourage participants to learn about and respect the diverse perspectives of others in relation to aspects of their work. The programme would need to develop the learning skills necessary to negotiate cross-cultural communication, to which both Leininger and Campinha-Bacote have drawn attention, and which were outlined earlier.

At the same time, any such programme needs to avoid the pitfalls of multiculturalist or transcultural models, which create an inappropriately narrow focus upon simplistic notions of culture and cultural differences (Stubbs, 1993; Culley, 1996; Gerrish *et al.*, 1996). These models have been based on the assumption that understanding one's own culture and the culture of others creates tolerance and respect for people from diverse backgrounds. Andrews and Boyle warn:

> the mere understanding of one's own culture and the culture of others is insufficient for the alleviation and potential eradication of prejudice, bigotry, racial, ethnic or cultural conflicts, discrimination or ethnoviolence. Rather, . . . health [care] providers must have positive experiences with members of other cultures and learn to value genuinely the contributions all cultures make to our multicultural society.
>
> (Andrews and Boyle, 1999: 15)

To continue to develop cultural competence and proficiency, the health practitioner needs to adopt an experiential approach to learning which results from sharing good practice within the organisation. Burford (1997) stresses that the learning process must be rethought, and redesigned, in order for there to be sufficient theoretical and educational background, within the context of placement experience, to support the novitiate health care worker in the stressful but also rewarding experiences of bicultural or transcultural interaction.

An integral part of achieving organisational change is the deployment of staff development processes in such a way as to support individual objectives, through appraisal and annual review, which take up cultural competencies as aspects of personal progression. Individual members of staff need to be aware of their responsibility in respecting differences, challenging discriminatory practices and at all times contributing to a healthy non-discriminatory organisational culture.

Evaluating culturally competent care

It is important that health care provision is regularly reviewed, monitored and evaluated to identify strengths and weaknesses in relation to cultural competence and proficiency. As a result of the health service reforms in the 1980s and 1990s the evaluation of the quality of care became 'a mandatory part of service provision' (Ellis and Whittington, 1993). It is essential that this be done against clearly identified indicators, targets and outcomes within identified timescales using a sophisticated framework: to establish what it is about the provision that works, and for whom; and to understand how and why it works (Connell and Kubisch, 1998; Weiss, 1985; Pawson and Tilley, 1997).

Different authors have identified outcomes of culturally competent care. These include Goode and Harrisone (2000), Bartol and Richardson (1998) and Ansari and Jackson (1995). For consumers, competence outcomes may include: increased self worth and self reliance; feelings of shared power with service providers; and higher levels of positive coping. For providers of services, outcomes may include the greater representation of staff from diverse backgrounds at all levels of the organisation, appropriate images of minority groups in training materials and the development of finesse in cultural assessments. Callister (2001) advises that the evaluation of culturally competent care should address both measurable and 'soft' outcomes to record the development process.

Conclusion

A person-centred, individualistic approach is important in providing culturally appropriate care. This approach avoids making assumptions about individual needs on the basis of any categorisation or ascribed characteristics of the individual concerned. Taking ethnicity as a marker of cultural identity, Gerrish et al. (1996) assert that specific ethnic identities must be located 'within their own particular social, political, economic and material contexts', as there is such a wide range within ethnic groups of 'access to and control over resources' that people with equally strong ethnic identities may differ widely in their ability to participate in the social life associated with forms of identity in a meaningful way. Practitioners need to be constantly vigilant to guard against the influence of stereotypes, which often takes away individuality from the care given to clients. A willingness to change one's own attitudes and demonstrate genuine interest in and appreciation of cultural differences, coupled with readiness to seek increased knowledge about the complex dimensions of culture, is essential to the provision of culturally competent care.

References

Ahmad, W. U. (ed.) (1993) *'Race' and Health in Contemporary Britain*, Buckingham: Open University Press.

Ahmad, W. U. and Atkin, K. (1996) ' "Race" and community care: an introduction', in Ahmad, W. U. and Atkin, K. (eds) (1996) *'Race' and Community Care*, Buckingham: Open University Press.

American Association of Medical Colleges (1984) 'Physicians in the twentieth century', in Kai, J. (ed.) (1999) *Valuing Diversity: A Resource for Effective Health Care of Ethnically Diverse Communities*, London: Royal College of General Practitioners.

Andrews, M. M. and Boyle, J. S. (1999) *Transcultural Concepts in Nursing Care*, New York: Lippincott.

Anionwu, E. (1996) 'Ethnic origin of sickle and thalassaemia counsellors: Does it matter?', in Kelleher, D. and Hillier, S. (eds) *Researching Cultural Differences in Health*, London: Routledge.

Ansari, K. H. and Jackson, J. (1995) *Managing Cultural Diversity at Work*, London: Kogan Page.

Bartol, G. M. and Richardson, L. (1998) 'Using literature to create cultural competence', *Journal of Nusing Scholarship*, vol. 30: 75–9.

Baxter, C. (1988) *Black Nurse: An Endangered Species*, London: National Extension College for Training in Health and Race.

Baxter, C. (1997) *Race Equality in Health Care Education*, London: Baillière Tindall.

Bharj, K. K. (1995) *Nurse Recruitment: An Asian Response*, Bradford: Race Relations. Research Unit, University of Bradford and Bradford and Ilkley Community College.

Braithwaite, R. L. Taylor, S. E. and Austin, J. N. (2000) *Building Health Coalitions in the Black Community*, London: Sage.

British Medical Association (1995) *Multicultural Health Care: Current Practice and Future Policy in Medical Education*, London: British Medical Association.

Buchan, J., Seccombe, I. J. and Smith, G. (1998) *Nurses Work: An Analysis of the UK Nursing Labour Market*, Aldershot: Ashgate.

Burford, B. (1997) *Cultural Competence: Myth, Useful Concept or Unattainable Goal? An Examination of the Human Resource Development Implications of Providing Healthcare in a Multi-cultural Community*, MBA Dissertation, University of Durham (unpublished).

Callister, L. C. (2001) 'Culturally competent care of women and newborns: knowledge, attitudes and skills', *Journal of Gynaecology and Neonatal Nursing*, vol. 30: 209–15.

Campinha-Bacote, J. (1988) 'Culturological assessment: an important factor in psychiatric consultation-liaison nursing', *Archives of Psychiatric Nursing*, vol. 2, no. 4.

Campinha-Bacote, J. (1994a) *The Process of Competence in Health Care: A Culturally Competent Model of Care*, Ohio: Transcultural C.A.R.E. Associates.

Campinha-Bacote, J. (1994b) 'Cultural competence in psychiatric mental health nursing', *Nursing Clinics of North America*, vol. 29, no. 1.

Castillo, H. M. (1996) 'Cultural diversity: implications for nursing', in Torres, S. (ed.) *Hispanic Voices*, New York: National League for Nursing Press.

Clinton, J. F. (1996) 'Cultural diversity and health care in America: knowledge fundamental to competence in baccalaureate nursing students', *Journal of Cultural Diversity*, vol. 3.

Cole, A. (1987) 'Racism in nursing', *Nursing Times*, vol. 78, no.18.

Collard, A. (1995) 'Training in racial harassment issues for community staff', *Nursing Times*, vol. 91 no. 2.

Commission for Racial Equality (CRE) (1976) Race Relations Act, London: Commission for Racial Equality.

Commission for Racial Equality (1995) *Annual Report of the Commission for Racial Equality*, London: Commission for Racial Equality.

Commission for Racial Equality (2000) Race Relations (Amendment) Act, London: Commission for Racial Equality.

Connell, J. P. and Kubisch, A. C. (1998) 'Applying a theory of change approach to the evaluation of comprehensive community initiatives: progress, prospects and problems', in Fulbright-Anderson, K., Kubisch, A. C. and Connell, J. P. (eds) *New Approaches to Evaluating Community Initiatives, Vol. 2 Theory, Measurement and Analysis*, Washington, DC: the Aspen Institute.

Cross, T., Bazron, B., Dennis, K. and Isaacs, M. (1989) *Towards a Culturally Competent System of Care: Vol. I*, Washington, DC: Georgetown University Child Development Centre, CASSP Technical Assistance Centre.

Crowe, M. (1996) 'Cancer nursing in Pakistan', *Journal of Cancer Care*, vol. 5, no. 4.

Culley, L. (1996) 'A critique of multiculturalism in health care: the challenge of nurse education', *Journal of Advanced Nursing*, vol. 23: 564–70.

Darr A. (1998) *Improving the Recruitment and Retention of Asian Students on Nursing, Midwifery, Radiography and Physiotherapy Courses: A Qualitative Research Study*, Bradford: University of Bradford.

Department of Health (DoH) (1993) *Report of a Working Party of the Standing Medical Advisory Committee on Sickle Cell, Thalasaemia and other Haemoglobinopathies*, London: HMSO.

Department of Health (1997) *The New NHS: Modern, Dependable*, London: Stationery Office.

Department of Health (1998a) *Our Healthier Nation: A Contract for Health – A Consultation Paper*, London: Stationery Office.

Department of Health (1998b) *Equal Opportunities and Monitoring in NHS Trusts*, London: Stationery Office.

Department of Health (1998c) *Tackling Racial Harassment in the NHS: A Plan for Action*, London: Stationery Office.

Department of Health (1998d) *Letting Through the Light*, London: Stationery Office.

Department of Health (1999) *Making a Difference. Strengthening the Nursing, Midwifery and Health Visiting Contribution to Health and Health Care*, London: Stationery Office.

Department of Health (2000a) *A Health Service of All Talents: Developing the NHS Workforce. Consultation Document on the Review of Workforce Planning*, London: Stationery Office.

Department of Health (2000b) *The Vital Connection: An Equalities Framework for the NHS. Working Together for Quality and Equality*, London: Department of Health.

Doyal, L., Hunt, G. and Mellor, J. (1980) *Migrant Workers in the NHS – Report of a Preliminary Survey*, London: Polytechnic of North London.

Ellis, R. and Whittington, D. (1993) *Quality Assurance in Health Care: A Handbook*, London: Edward Arnold.

English National Board for Nursing, Midwifery and Health Visiting (ENB) (1996) 'The evaluation of pre-registration undergraduate degrees in nursing and midwifery', *Research Highlights*, London: English National Board.

English National Board for Nursing, Midwifery and Health Visiting (1998) 'Recruiting minority ethnic groups into nursing, midwifery and health visiting', *Research Report Series* no. 7, London: English National Board.

Esmail, A. and Everington, S. (1993) 'Racial discrimination against doctors from ethnic minorities', *British Medical Journal*, vol. 306: 619–92.

Fernando, S. (1991) *Mental Health, Race and Culture*, Basingstoke: Macmillan.

Freedman, L. P. (2000) 'Human rights and women's health', in Goldman, M. B. and Hatch, M. C. (eds) *Women and Health*, New York: Guildford.

French, S., Watters, D. and Mathews, D. (1994) 'Nursing as a career choice for women in Pakistan', *Journal of Advanced Nursing*, vol. 19, no. 1.

Gerrish, K., Husband, C. and McKenzie, J. (1996) *Nursing for a Multi-ethnic Society*, Buckingham: Open University Press.

Gill, P. S. and Green, P. (1996) 'Learning for a multicultural society', *British Journal of General Practice*, vol. 19, no. 96.

Goode, T. (2000) *Promoting Cultural Diversity and Cultural Competence*, Washington, DC: Georgetown University Child Development Center – National Center for Cultural Competence.

Goode, T. and Harrisone, S. (2000) *Cultural Competence in Primary Health Care: Partnerships for a Research Agenda*, Washington, DC: Georgetown University Child Development Center – National Center for Cultural Competence.

Hastings-Asatourian, B. (2000) *Gatekeeping Inequity*, Bradford: Race Relations Research Unit, Bradford University and Bradford & Ilkley College.

Hicks, C. (1982a) 'Racism in nursing', *Nursing Times*, vol. 78, no. 18: 743–44.

Hicks, C. (1982b) 'Racism in nursing', *Nursing Times*, vol. 78, no. 18: 789–92.

Im, E., Meleis, A. I. and Lee, K. A. (1999) 'Cultural competence of measurement scales of menopausal symptoms: use in research among Korean women', *International Journal of Nursing Studies*, vol. 36, no. 6.

Jennings-Dozier, K. (1999) 'Predicting intentions to obtain a Pap smear among African American and Latina women: testing the theory of planned behaviour', *Nursing Research*, vol. 48, no.4.

Jones, F.C. (1999) 'Cultural influences', in Broome, M. E. and Rollins, J. A. (eds) *Core Curriculum for the Nursing Care of Children and their Families*, New York: Janetti.

Kai, J. (ed.) (1999) *Valuing Diversity: A Resource for Effective Health Care of Ethnically Diverse Communities*, London: Royal College of General Practitioners.

Lee-Cunin, M. (1989) *Daughters of Seacole*, Batley: West Yorkshire Low Pay Unit.

Leininger, M. (1995) *Transcultural Nursing: Concepts, Theories, Research and Practices*, New York: McGraw-Hill.

Lester, N. (1998) 'Cultural competence: a nursing dialogue', *American Journal of Nursing*, vol. 98: 26–33.

Lipson, J. and Steiger, N. (1996) *Self Care in a Multicultural Context*, Thousand Oaks, CA: Sage.

McGee, P. (2000) *Culturally-Sensitive Nursing Care: A Critique*, Unpublished Ph.D. thesis, University of Central England, Birmingham.

Mares, P., Henley, A. and Baxter, C. (1985) *Healthcare in Multicultural Britain*, London: National Extension College for Training in Health and Race/Health Education Council.

Meleis, A. I. (1996) 'Culturally competent scholarship: substance and rigour', *Advanced Nursing Science*, vol. 19, no.1.

NHS Executive (1994) *Code of Practice: Equal Opportunities in Employment*, London: HMSO.

Nursing Council of New Zealand (1996) *Guidelines for Cultural Safety Component in Nursing and Midwifery Education*, Auckland: Nursing Council of New Zealand.

Papps, E. and Ramsden, I. (1996) 'Cultural safety in nursing: the New Zealand experience', *International Journal for Quality in Health Care*, vol. 8, no. 5.

Pawson, R. and Tilley, N. (1997) *Realistic Evaluation*, London: Sage.

Pearson, M. (1987) 'Racism: the great divide', *Nursing Times*, vol. 83, no. 24.

Platzer, H. (1988) 'Redressing the balance', *Nursing Standard*, vol. 2, no. 15.

Poulton, J., Rylance, G. W. and Johnson, M. R. D. (1986) 'Medical teaching of the cultural aspects of ethnic minorities: does it exist?' *Medical Education*, vol. 20: 492–7.

Rashid, A. (1990) 'Asian doctors and nurses in the NHS', in McAvoy, B. and Donaldson, L., *Health Care for Asians*, Oxford: Oxford University Press.

Sashidharan, S. P. and Francis, E. (1993) 'Epidemiology, ethnicity and schizophrenia', in Ahmad, W. U. (ed.) *Race and Health in Contemporary Britain*. Buckingham: Open University Press.

Smith, L. S. (1998) 'Concept analysis: cultural competence', *Journal of Cultural Diversity*, vol. 5: 4–10.

Stenhouse, G. H. and Pemberton, J. D. (1999) 'Learning and knowledge management in the intelligent organisation', *Participation & Empowerment: An International Journal*, vol. 7, no. 5.

Stubbs, P. (1993) 'Ethnically-sensitive or anti-racist? Models for health research and service delivery', in Ahmad, W. U. (ed.) *Race and Health in contemporary Britain*, Buckingham: Open University Press.

Thorpe, D. E. and Baker, C. P. (1995) 'Addressing "cultural competence" in health-care education', *Paediatric Physical Therapy*, vol. 14, no. 3.

Torkington, P. (1987) 'Sorry, wrong colour', *Nursing Times*, vol. 83, no. 24.

University of Central England, Faculty of Health and Community Care (2001) *Recruitment and Retention in Nursing and Professions Allied to Medicine of Individuals from Black and Minority Ethnic Communities*, Final Report, Birmingham: University of Central England.

United Kingdom Central Council for Nursing, Midwifery and Health Visiting (UKCC) (1999) *Fitness for Practice: The UKCC Commission for Nursing and Midwifery Education*, London: United Kingdom Central Council for Nursing Midwifery and Health Visiting.

Weiss, C. H. (1995) 'Nothing as practical as good theory: exploring theory-based evaluation for comprehensive community initiatives for children and families', in Connell, J. P., Kubisch, A. C., Schorr, L. B. and Weiss, C. H. (eds) *New Approaches to Evaluating Community Initiatives: Concepts, Methods and Contexts*, Washington, DC: The Aspen Institute.

Wells, S. A. (1995) 'Creating a culturally competent workforce', *Caring Magazine*, December: 50–3.

Willis, W. O. (1999) 'Culturally competent nursing care during perinatal period', *Journal of Perinatal and Neonatal Nursing*, vol. 13, no. 3.

Woodley Team Support (1995) *Report of the Independent Review Panel to East London and City Health Authority and Newham Council*, London: East London and City Health Authority.

Chapter 8

Disability and oppression

Changing theories and practices

Geoffrey Mercer

Introduction

The theory and practice of disability became increasingly contested through the last quarter of the twentieth century. The public, professional and policy perception was that it constituted a 'personal tragedy', with disabled people the unfortunate victims of their impairment, directed to a lifetime of 'care' and dependency. However, this individual perspective attracted growing criticism from emerging organisations of disabled people and disability activists. These critics highlighted the wide-ranging discrimination experienced by disabled people and developed a theoretical analysis in which disability is defined as a form of social exclusion and oppression. Political campaigns called for a 'rights not charity' approach.

This scenario seems tailor-made for the application of anti-oppressive social work. And yet it has been disabled people and their allies who have taken the initiative in raising disability issues – often in the face of concerted opposition or general indifference from policy makers, academics and service providers. This chapter will address this apparent contradiction. It will: first, outline the development of a 'social model' to replace the individual approach to disability; second, explore existing social service provision for disabled clients; and third, examine attempts by disabled people and organisations controlled by them to develop radical new initiatives to promote the inclusion of disabled people, with particular reference to 'independent living'.

From individual to social model of disability

In modern times, the dominant approach to disability has equated it with long-term sickness and incapacity (World Health Organisation, 1980). This diagnostic focus on individual defects and limitations associated with disabled bodies and minds is located in medical knowledge, which in turn provides the rationale for medical and allied interventions. The aim has been cure, rehabilitation and care. In health and social policy terms this dictates that disabled people must accept their dependence on others, whether professional experts or informal family carers. More widely, it rationalises the limited participation if not exclusion of the 'person with a disability' from everyday social life.

For critics, this 'personal tragedy', or individual and in modern times heavily medicalised approach, has dominated policy thinking and practice with respect to disability (Oliver, 1990). In response, disabled people have campaigned against the injustice of their second-class status in contemporary society with gathering intensity. They have also contested the orthodox view that impairment causes an individual's removal from, or marginalisation in, the mainstream of society. In Britain, a key contribution to these early debates was provided by the Union of the Physically Impaired Against Segregation (UPIAS). Its *Fundamental Principles of Disability* manifesto differentiated 'impairment' from 'disability' in a novel way:

> *impairment* is defined as lacking of part or all of a limb, or having a defective limb, organ or mechanism of the body; whereas
> *disability* is the disadvantage or restriction of activity caused by a contemporary social organisation which takes little or no account of people who have physical impairments and thus excludes them from participation in the mainstream of social activities.
>
> (UPIAS, 1976: 14)

This formulation was subsequently extended to cover all impairments (Oliver, 1990). As an example, the inability to see constitutes visual impairment, while the failure to provide information in accessible formats for visually impaired people constitutes disability. UPIAS broadly accepted the medical designation of impairment, but overturned the orthodox view of disability. It sought to draw a clear line between areas of medical and social concern. The UPIAS statement does not claim that all the problems of social exclusion are attributable to the individual's impairment, and does not reject the importance of appropriate medical intervention. Instead, it espouses a 'relational' definition of disability that accentuates the reduced opportunities to participate in society that confront people with an impairment because of social, environmental and cultural barriers (Finkelstein, 1980, 1991). From this perspective, the analytical and political spotlight is directed at the 'disabling society' rather than the individual's impairment.

This focus on the social dimensions to disability has been further elaborated into a wide-ranging 'social model' approach by theorists such as Mike Oliver (1983, 1990) and Paul Abberley (1987). They have stressed the analysis of disability as a form of social oppression that demonstrates considerable historical and cultural variation. In Western societies, the rise of industrial capitalism created powerful trends towards the exclusion of disabled people from mainstream society. Disabled people were increasingly identified as a social problem, leading to their stigmatisation as individuals unable to make a full contribution to economic and social life. An emerging policy response saw their growing segregation in residential institutions such as workhouses, asylums and special schools, and reliance on state welfare, informal care and public charity. For disability critics, the aim was to theorise disability as a key line of social division and exclusion comparable to sexism, racism and ageism (Abberley, 1987).

Although there had been many critiques of the medicalisation of health and social care, these had rarely been extended to the individualised and medicalised approach to disability (Barnes and Mercer, 1996). It was only at the behest of disabled people that a socio-political analysis of disability gained momentum. Its starting point is the claim that: 'it is society which disabled physically impaired people' (UPIAS, 1976: 3). The supporting evidence is found in the wide-ranging discrimination practised against disabled people in respect of education, employment, leisure activities, transport, housing, income and wealth, family life and reproduction, abuse and violence and their reinforcement in media and wider cultural representations (Finkelstein, 1980; Oliver 1983, 1990; Barnes, 1991). This amounts to a pattern of systematic exclusion against disabled people.

Nevertheless, the 'social model' does not constitute a comprehensive theory of the social oppression experienced by disabled people. Initially, in Britain, it was given a neo-Marxist formulation, but it has been influenced by a widening range of theoretical standpoints, most particularly feminist and anti-racist analyses and more recently by post-structuralist and post-modernist accounts (Barnes *et al.*, 1999).

Like any social protest movement of recent times, disabled people do not all 'sing from the same hymn sheet'. This applies as much to support for a socio-political analysis of disability, as self-identification as a disabled person. The disabled population is extremely diverse in terms of social class, age, gender, sexuality, ethnicity and 'race', and too little attention had been paid to the ways in which disability interacts with these other social divisions, just as feminist and anti-racist analyses have been taken to task for ignoring disabled women and disabled black people. The early emphasis on the common experience of oppression that unites disabled people has also given way to a greater recognition that the disabled population includes people with a diverse range of impairments and contrasting experiences (Morris, 1991).

In addition, the early social model writers concentrated so heavily on the social construction of disability that they ignored the extent to which impairment is itself socially located and interpreted. For example, those who designate themselves as 'mental health system users/survivors' often reject the presumption of impairment as a medical diagnosis. Again, people with learning difficulties have felt excluded from disabled people's organisations and politics because of its primary focus on disabled bodies rather than minds.

Service provision for disabled people

British disability policy has consistently exemplified a personal tragedy approach, by stressing individual care ('special needs') over collective needs, segregation over inclusion, and charity over civil rights (Oliver, 1990; Finkelstein, 1991). The service orientation has been dominated by approaches fixed in notions of medical cure, care and rehabilitation, reinforced by psychological approaches to coping with 'loss'.

This forms part of a detailed criticism of the professional domination of services for disabled people. Professionals represent a diverse range of vested interests 'servicing' disabled people – what amounts to a veritable 'disability business' (Albrecht, 1992). Crucially, they dominate the form and character of the helper–helped relationship. This includes perception of disabled people's needs and the appropriateness and quality of services (Oliver, 1983). Far from adopting an 'enabling' agenda, health and social care professionals are identified as part of the problem not part of the solution to disability. From a social oppression perspective, a fundamental reformulation of the helper–helped relationship is necessary. This entails a transformation of the professional's role from managing the disabled client to becoming a resource in supporting disabled people to achieve their own goals (Finkelstein, 1981).

Oliver and Sapey's (1999: 60) summary critique of the organisation of social work focuses on three main issues. First, that social workers act as arbiters of need between disabled people and the state. Second, that the responsibilities for services to disabled people were uncoordinated and distributed between a large number of organisations and rehabilitation professions. Third, the services that were available tended to reflect the professional interests and aspirations of those workers rather than being based on any analysis of disability and the needs of disabled people.

The typical location for service delivery was large impersonal bureaucratic organisations, that were routinely required to ration scarce resources among competing demands or needs. The multiplicity of professionals actually or potentially involved with disabled clients creates its own uncertainties about which professional to deal with, or which service agency (Wilding, 1982). It has not helped that social work with disabled clients has carried a low status (Barclay Committee, 1982), or that services for disabled people have been accorded a low priority (Sapey and Hewitt, 1991).

The place of residential services has been central to conflicts between disabled people and health and social care professionals. It is little coincidence that so much of the early political mobilisation of disabled people centred on activists' opposition to institutional life. It was characterised by a loss of freedom, choice, close personal relationships and privacy (Hunt, 1966). In the stark terms adopted by Eric Miller and Geraldine Gwynne (1972) the lives of inmates are regulated by a 'warehousing' approach. This is because their future is regarded as akin to 'social death'. While a more liberal 'horticultural' model of residential care is acknowledged, this was regarded as misplaced or misleading because it suggested a capacity for independence and capacity for 'growth' among disabled residents that was not achievable. This provider-led approach to service provision meant that the crucial decisions about what was in the disabled person's best interest were made by non-disabled experts.

Nevertheless, in the final decades of the twentieth century criticism built up over the perceived shortcomings and failures of existing services for disabled people. These included: the over-reliance on and impact of segregated institutions; an over-emphasis on regulation and control; low standards/outcomes; the abuse and neglect of inmates; and little public accountability (Oliver and Barnes, 1998).

Changing policy agenda

Statutory agencies, such as local authorities, must act within the existing legislative and general political climate. The last quarter of the twentieth century is notable for the growth in 'New Right' policies that called for a retrenchment in state expenditure, with social programmes a primary target, not least because they also encouraged dependence on the welfare state. In contrast with such programmes, the New Right proposed a much more significant role for market mechanisms, private and voluntary initiatives in welfare and a return to strong family values and individual responsibility. At the same time, this period witnessed the emergence of campaigns organised around 'social welfare' groups, including an increasingly active disabled people's movement. It argued for equal citizenship and civil rights and a re-think on service support for disabled people.

Despite their very different political standpoints, both New Right policies and disabled people's organisations promoted the merits of user involvement in service provision (Oliver and Barnes, 1998). The Chronically Sick and Disabled Person's Act 1970 suggested an important shift towards a more service-led approach by involving disabled people in their planning and delivery. The 'discovery of service users' was also recognised in debates within social welfare professions about working in more participatory ways (Beresford and Croft, 1993).

However, debates about user involvement became a battleground between the conflicting aims and interpretations of the service system and the disabled people's movement. In general terms, there has been a clash between the more 'consumerist' views adhered to in the state and welfare system, and the more 'democratic' interpretation espoused by disabled people's organisations.

These trends and tensions are well-illustrated by the policy embrace of 'normalisation'. Normalisation centred on enabling disabled people to lead 'ordinary' lives by enjoying greater opportunities for choice, self-realisation and independence (Wolfensberger, 1972). Four key features of this policy are: (1) it is concerned to ensure that services and service delivery systems are responsive to the variety of individual need; (2) it has an emphasis on citizenship as implying a set of rights which extend to people with special needs, including the right to involvement in decisions about the life styles and choices open to them; (3) it sees the disabled person's involvement in decision making as both an end in itself and also as a means to an end of personal growth and development; and (4) in stressing the importance of gaining access to 'ordinary life styles', it implies an increasing role for mainstream services such as housing, leisure, education and employment at the expense of specialised – and often segregated – residential and day services (Wistow and Barnes, 1993: 283).

Government enthusiasm for market led private and voluntary sector initiatives was influenced by claims that the most successful private companies are those that listen to their customers and highlight the importance of quality issues generally (Pollitt, 1990). Consumer needs and preferences became a management tool to enhance the quality of service provision, and company profitability. When used by the public sector, they were also promoted as making a reality of accountability and citizenship rights – further reinforced by the growth of 'Citizen Charters' (Clarke and Stewart, 1992). Thus, implementation of user involvement in the public and voluntary sectors highlighted a 'weaker' rather than a 'stronger' version of consumerism. In the case of normalisation and service policy for people with learning difficulties, there was little evidence of a commitment to 'empower users in decision-making about the design, management, delivery and review of services' (Wistow and Barnes, 1993: 285).

Indeed, from a social model perspective, the stress given to the participation of this impairment group in 'socially valued life styles' more accurately expressed a professional's vision of what services should be like for people with learning difficulties. The old power relationships were perpetuated despite the move from long-stay institutions to the community: 'normalisation enabled professionals . . . to maintain a key role in community care and adapt to new services by developing new models of practice' (Chappell, 1997: 48). A further contradiction of normalisation as a policy for user involvement is that it was premised on an analysis that identified people with learning difficulties as 'the problem' and their lifestyles as lacking value or authenticity. This clash of views is vividly illustrated in the failure of day care centres to 'enable' independent living (Barnes, 1990).

For disabled activists, the emphasis had to move on so that user-involvement encompassed user-led if not user-controlled services and support. New encouragement was provided by subsequent legislative changes, such as the Disabled Persons Act 1986, the National Health Service and Community Care Act 1990, and the Community Care (Direct Payments)

Act 1996. The implementation of needs-led care assessment set down in the Disabled Persons Act 1986 and given central billing in the community care policy framework developed in the late 1980s and early 1990s, had as one of the main aims to bring the user (and carer) into decisions surrounding care management and assessment. However the representation of official policy and experience at the local level often clashed. Surveys of disabled people reported that 'delays, lack of information, poor communication, patronising attitudes and a lack of collaborative working were commonplace' (Priestley, 1998: 661).

This was typified by the complaint that the process of needs assessment was itself disabling because it continued in an individualistic and medicalised mode. Although there has always been some scope for the applications of a 'social work imagination', service practice has generally found it lacking (Sapey and Hewitt, 1991: 42). Hence, disabled people's organisations represented the community care reforms as more a threat than an encouragement to social inclusion. Morris conceptualises this in the following way:

> A political and ideological battle is being waged . . . between government and national disability organisations, between social service authorities and local disability organisations, and, most importantly, within the daily lives of disabled individuals . . . The terrain of this battle is . . . named 'community care'.
>
> (Morris, 1993: ix)

The Disability Discrimination Act (DDA) 1995 and the establishment of the Disability Rights Commission in 2000 herald further changes in the wider disability policy context. It was grudgingly acknowledged that the denial of equal rights to disabled people was morally and politically unacceptable, although two decades later than comparable action in respect of sexism and racism. Yet despite the Equal Opportunities Commission's conclusion that the DDA is perhaps 'the most radical of discrimination laws' (EOR, 1996: 31), its reception among disabled people's organisations has been more muted because of the number of 'escape clauses' it contains (Bagilhole, 1997). The Human Rights Act 1998 adds a further dimension to disabled people's campaigns but overall disabled people have been left feeling that much more has been promised than actually delivered in challenging their social oppression.

Disabled people's initiatives

The growth in user-controlled organisations allied to a social model analysis has encouraged new models of policy development. It has involved campaigns for consciousness raising and the promotion and control of services to support independent living within a democratic and accountable organisation (Campbell and Oliver, 1996).

Consciousness raising

A feature of the politicisation of disabled people has been its engagement with diverse groups of disabled people (with physical/sensory impairments, mental health system users/survivors, and people with learning difficulties). This is confirmed in the rise of self-advocacy among people with learning difficulties from the initial, tentative moves towards user participation in the 1970s (Goodley, 2000). Its history amply demonstrates the general unease and frequent opposition of service providers, as well as parental and carer-dominated groups, to user-involvement (Shearer, 1972, 1973). Significantly, the first 'People First' self-advocacy group that was established in London in 1984 located itself separately from a service base.

A further important contribution to the politicisation of disabled people has been the emergence of Disability Equality Training (DET) courses. These centre on elaborating a social barriers perspective to disability (Gillespie-Sells and Campbell, 1991). Indeed, through the 1990s a national network of DET trainers, disability consultants, and organisations of and for disabled people have been marketing DET (or similar) courses to schools, colleges, businesses, voluntary organisations and charities, as well as in places where disabled people are congregated such as day centres and residential institutions.

Although lagging well behind 'race' and gender equality training (Dalrymple and Burke, 1995), it was possible for disability trainers to build on the experience of these other groups. Even so, there remained some opposition among both public and private sector organisations to disabled people taking the lead in this activity. Disabled organisations recognised that having an impairment is a necessary but not a sufficient condition for becoming an effective DET trainer. This resulted in the establishment of a Trainers Forum for disabled people that gradually built up a pool of qualified trainers. Initially these were concentrated in the London area but DET soon became a central activity offered by Centres for Independent Living (CILs) and Coalitions of Disabled People around England, Scotland and Wales. While not the primary stimulus, DET training sponsored a wider involvement of individual disabled people in political campaigns against 'disabling' barriers and attitudes.

Moves towards independent or integrated living

The focus on independent living by disabled people extends across developments in Europe and North America (DeJong, 1979). In Britain, CILs took off in the early 1980s. There was no single CIL model, but they comprised organisations controlled and largely run by disabled people that provided a range of peer support services.

Derbyshire Centre for Integrated Living (DCIL) became Britain's first such organisation. It took a vanguard role in designing and delivering services based on a social model approach that broke down the professional 'knowledge monopoly'. It engaged disabled people as primary actors in developing a support system of services for integrated living that contrasted sharply with traditional (segregated) modes of service provision. DCIL based its system of community support on seven key needs and priorities identified by disabled people (information, environmental access, housing, technical aids and assistance, personal assistance, counselling and peer support, and transport) (Davis and Mullender, 1993). These arose directly from experience in running the Grove Road independent living experiment – as an escape route from institutional life (Davis, 1981). Disabled people's groups have explored a variety of housing and community support schemes more recently – including housing associations, lifetime homes and trust initiatives.

As an illustration, access to information and advice has been highlighted by disabled people as fundamental to inclusion in contemporary society – something denied by mainstream providers. The 1970 Chronically Sick and Disabled Persons Act required all local authorities to provide appropriate information about their services for disabled people, and this was reinforced by the Disabled Persons Act 1986. However, it was the establishment of the National Association of Disablement Information and Advice Services in 1978, now known as the Disablement Information and Advice Line (DIAL), that made most headway with disabled people (Davis and Woodward, 1981). This service aimed to provide general 'disability' information as well as materials geared to specific groups within the disabled population. The areas covered span accessible housing, technical aids and equipment, benefits, employment opportunities, disability organisations, disability arts and culture. Nevertheless, provision still remains very uneven across the country, with a lack of resources and inadequate services in key areas.

The above examples demonstrate the way in which CILs have been central to the implementation of disabled people's distinctive philosophy of independent living. As Priestley (1999: 166) comments, these organisations 'provide living models of the way in which disabled people can be effectively engaged in all aspects of welfare production – as individual consumers, exercising choice through self-assessment and self-management; as advocates, providing peer support and positive role modelling; as representatives, contributing to the strategic development and evaluation of service design; as participative citizens, seeking to identify and remove disabling barriers in their communities; as political actors, within a wider movement for social change'.

However, such opportunities remain contingent on a variety of factors at the local level, including the commitment to user participation, the political agenda and the level of organisation among disabled people. In practice, even sympathetic local authorities sometimes balked at the prospect of CILs replacing existing service provision because they smacked of privatisation and an attack on public accountability (Priestley, 1999). At the same time, it is important to recognise the contribution of parallel initiatives outside CILs, for example, in self-help organisations of disabled people, such as the Spinal Injuries Association (D'Aboville, 1991).

Overall, the administrative and provider focus on care, individualism and segregated services have been opposed by disabled people's demands for citizenship rights, equality and participation. The moves towards integrated living outcomes and the removal of social barriers moved slowly, but in places significantly, forward. CILs have been a major catalyst in ensuring that disabled people's own perception of what will improve their quality of life is accorded a higher priority. Nevertheless, enhancing services is one important contribution to a wider political agenda of full citizenship rights, which demands much wider social changes (Barnes, 1991; Morris, 1994; Priestley, 1999).

Direct payments

The growth of self-managed personal assistance schemes dates from the early 1980s. A key initiative to taking the independent living route originated in Hampshire. Some disabled residents of the local 'Le Court' Cheshire Home persuaded the local authority to transfer funding for their institutional care into support provision in the community. At the time, the National Assistance Act of 1948 prohibited local authorities from making cash payments directly to disabled people. However, nationally CILs and transfer funding arrangements developed slowly in the 1980s, with local authorities uncertain about their cost and legality, and wary of losing control of service provision.

It was the Conservative Government's establishment of the Independent Living Fund (ILF) in 1988 that marked an important boost to self-managed personal assistance schemes. The aim was to help disabled people to live outside residential homes and to have greater control of their service support. Although ILF was formally ended by the implementation of the NHS and Community Care Act 1990, its popularity among disabled people led to its continuation in two guises: an Extension Fund (to maintain payments to original recipients), and the 93 Fund (for new applicants, on slightly different terms). What the ILF had demonstrated was that self-managed personal support was a realistic and popular option (Kestenbaum, 1993; Morris, 1993).

Meanwhile, the British Council of Disabled People (BCODP) orchestrated a national campaign for direct payments. Commissioned research demonstrated that self-managed support packages were 30–40 per cent cheaper than equivalent statutory services (Zarb and Nadash, 1994). The study also confirmed that disabled people expressed higher levels of satisfaction with these support systems because of the greater levels of control, choice and flexibility generated. With widening political support, including from the Association of Directors of Social Services, the Community Care (Direct Payments) Act 1996 legalised direct payments from April 1997. Anyone aged over 18 who is assessed by a local authority as needing community care services and who is deemed 'willing and able' to manage payments becomes eligible. The social work task of assessing need remains but the role of purchasing services and employing personal assistants is ceded to the disabled person, so breaking down the traditional helper–helped relationship.

Self-managed support schemes cover both direct and indirect payments: in the latter the cash payments are administered by a third party such as a local disabled people's organisation, trust or other agent on behalf of the disabled person. Self-management of direct payments covers a range of financial and employment responsibilities including legal, insurance, health and safety issues. It is a complex and daunting task, particularly for individuals who have traditionally been treated as passive and dependent, and far from all local authorities have in place an adequate advice and support service (Zarb and Nadash, 1994). It is here that CILs have played an invaluable role in supporting disabled people. Nevertheless, studies report that some groups, such as older disabled people prefer a third party arrangement (Payne et al., 1998), while innovative trust funds are a recommended option for people with learning difficulties (Holman and Bewley, 1999; Ryan, 1999). Conversely, black disabled people have been discouraged from the direct payments route because some professionals presume that they are supported by a strong family network (Bignall, 2000).

In February 2000, direct payments were made available to people aged 65 and over and the New Labour Government has expressed its commitment to ensure that all local authorities operate direct payments schemes. The Carers and Disabled Children Act (2000) further extends these schemes to disabled 16- and 17-year-olds and to parents of disabled children. This wider availability of direct payments highlights the need for greater flexibility in the service support available and its mode of delivery (Kestenbaum, 1996).

Nevertheless, direct payments have not overcome long-standing grievances, particularly over the refusal to concede self-assessment, while the strict monitoring procedures and excessive bureaucracy also attract criticism (Kestenbaum, 1996). There is also a low ceiling for cash payments, and the progress towards increasing the number of groups eligible to participate in the scheme has been a major frustration for disabled people. This ties in with a general lack of evidence of concerted efforts to develop innovative models of management consistent with user-led services (Begum and

Gillespie-Sells, 1994). Moreover, the Community Care (Direct Payments) Act 1996 is not mandatory and this has resulted in its uneven implementation across the country. A recent survey suggested that less than 30 per cent of local authorities in the North of England, Northern Ireland and Wales provide direct payments. In contrast, 70 per cent of authorities in London, South West England and Scotland provide direct payments (JRF, 2000). More positively, the new legislation led to the establishment of the National Centre for Independent Living (NCIL) in 1996 to provide training and advice to encourage the development of direct/indirect payment schemes.

The contrasting ways in which value conflicts have been played out between the competing philosophies of community care and independent/integrated living has been closely documented by Mark Priestley (1998, 1999). He illustrates how CIL users in Derbyshire experience the continuation of traditional, individualistic care assessment by social workers in broadly negative ways. By contrast, self-assessment gives a crucial stimulus to the self-empowerment of disabled service users. The degree of financial support provided is obviously crucial, since otherwise the 'difficult decisions' over resource allocation are simply devolved to service users (Priestley, 1999). Overall, the participation of disabled people in managing their own affairs marks an important advance in challenging established cultural values about the dependency of disabled people in society. It has been the growth of user-led organisations that has been the catalyst for pioneering new roles for disabled people, whether managing a self-support scheme or acting as 'peer advocate' or 'integrated living advisor' for disabled people. Such initiatives combine self-help, peer support and political change in novel ways (Barnes et al., 2000).

The continued move towards user-led services presumes some combination of the following: more support for personal development, and general development of skills, including DET; practical support for community living, whether through self-managed personal assistance or DCIL's 'seven needs'; adequate, secure funding of independent organisations of disabled people; and equal opportunities – in both access and support – across the disabled population (Beresford and Croft, 1993).

Some concern has been generated by moves towards more strict means testing of support income, while future policy on charging for home care and non-residential social services carries further financial threats to disabled people. The Government's proposals for joined-up governance go some way forward in stressing the role of citizens rather than consumers in shaping service development and accountability. New trusts merging health and social services may become involved in the provision of independent living services, but exactly how is uncertain. To empower disabled people means tackling the broad range of barriers that they confront. If action is to be taken against the causes of disability rather than its symptoms a broad anti-disablism strategy is required that builds on anti-oppressive practice in social services but goes well beyond its organisational boundaries. As yet disabled people's priorities have not been embedded, while social work and social care values have an uncertain status in the new system.

Identifying a new social work role

A Central Council for Education and Training in Social Work (CCETSW, 1974) report listed a number of possible reforms but these had no input from organisations of disabled people. A decade later, the Barclay Report (Barclay Committee, 1982) outlined the importance of social care planning, community social work and counselling, but again this seemed at odds with the demands by disabled people for supporting independent living. More recently the British Association of Social Workers (BASW) (1990) and the Central Council for Education and Training in Social Work have given further consideration to working with disabled clients. CCETSW's report *Disability Issues: Developing Anti-Discriminatory Practice* (Stevens, 1991) actually aligns itself with a social model approach although this is rather submerged in a concern for the development of a competence-based vocational qualification rather than a redefinition of the social work task. CCETSW has also stressed issues such as participation, empowerment and choice even if the overt embrace of anti-oppressive practice remains contentious in the social work curriculum (Wilson and Beresford, 2000).

The paradox is that a burgeoning anti-oppressive theory and research focus in the social work literature has followed a separate and different trajectory to its incorporation in disability theory and organisations of disabled people. It is only in the last decade that disability has acquired a significant presence in standard social work texts (Dominelli, 1998). Even then, anti-oppressive theory remains distanced from disability issues, with few applications to disabled clients. There is also a failure to bridge the gap between social work and disability research. Although the latter constitutes a further dimension to exploring the social exclusion of disabled people, it has attracted relatively little attention in the social work literature on anti-oppressive practice until very recently (Dalrymple and Burke, 1995).

An emphasis on disability equality training in social work education would be a starting point. It brings a challenge to traditional, medicalised notions of normality, or established 'solutions' such as residential care. Social work in general has yet to implement the right of disabled people to choose their own support services that will facilitate integrated/independent living options. The promotion of such services demands a range of skills of negotiation, assessment, advocacy and counselling. Yet again the wider goal of social inclusion for disabled people must be maintained. Hitherto, counselling of disabled people, if accepted as part of the social work role, has been to help people cope with or come to terms with 'their disability' rather than promoting an enabling social model perspective, or recognising the expertise and preferences of disabled people.

A further dimension to user-involvement arises from suggestions that this should extend to participation in defining and developing standards for professional practice (Harding and Beresford, 1996). While service users now have some involvement in the education and training of social work and social care students and practitioners, this has not yet been developed in any systematic, coherent or sustained way (Shennan, 1998). Consequently, the power to define what constitutes anti-oppressive practice (or theory) remains with practice teachers, tutors and other academics, rather than service users or students (Wilson and Beresford, 2000). Nevertheless, there has been a move among social work academics and practitioners to concede disabled service users' knowledge and expertise in relation to their own oppression (Dominelli, 1998). Disability theorists, on the other hand, sometimes presume a level of politicisation across the disabled community that is not generally confirmed in social work experience.

Conclusion

The rise of the disabled people's movement has triggered a wide-ranging critique of traditional approaches to disability as a personal tragedy. The elaboration of a radical, alternative that approaches disability as a form of social oppression has redirected attention away from the dominant professional and service focus on an individual's impairment. Instead, the source of disability is located in the range of social barriers that inhibit and prevent disabled people's inclusion in mainstream society. This shift in disability theory has been complemented by innovative attempts to transform service provision to enable disabled people to live more independently in the community.

In both theoretical and practice terms, disability writings demonstrate clear overlaps with anti-oppressive writings in social work. Yet, the experience of disabled people and organisations controlled by them, has been that social work has not attempted, at least until very recently, to engage with criticisms of its failure to confront disability issues. There remains a disappointing reluctance on the part of social work theory and practice to move away from rather traditional individualistic and medicalised approaches to disability. This extends to recognition of the initiatives promoted by organisations of disabled people in developing qualitatively different types of service support.

The story of the last quarter of the twentieth century is that, insofar as disabled people have been empowering themselves, they have received scant support or comfort from service providers generally and social workers in particular, not least those arguing for anti-oppressive practice.

References

Abberley, P. (1987) 'The concept of oppression and the development of a social theory of disability', *Disability, Handicap and Society*, vol. 2, no. 1.

Aboville, d', E. (1991) 'Social Work in an organisation of disabled people', in Oliver, M. (ed.) *Social Work, Disabled People and Disabling Environments*, London: Jessica Kingsley.

Albrecht, G. L. (1992) *The Disability Business*, London: Sage.

Bagilhole, B. (1997) *Equal Opportunities and Social Policy*, London: Longman.

Barclay Committee (1982) *Social Workers: Their Role and Tasks*, London: Bedford Square Press.

Barnes, C. (1990), *Cabbage Syndrome: The Social Construction of Dependence*, London: Falmer.

Barnes, C. (1991), *Disabled People in Britain and Discrimination: A Case for Anti-Discrimination Legislation*, London: Hurst.

Barnes, C. (ed.) (1993) *Making Our Own Choices*, Belper: British Council of Disabled People.

Barnes, C. and Mercer, G. (eds) (1996) *Exploring the Divide: Illness and Disability*, Leeds: The Disability Press.

Barnes, C., Mercer, G. and Morgan, H. (2000) *Creating Independent Futures: Stage One Report*, Leeds: The Disability Press.

Barnes, C., Mercer, G. and Shakespeare, T. (1999) *Exploring Disability*, Cambridge: Polity Press.

Begum, N. and Gillespie-Sells, K. (1994) *Towards Managing User-Led Services*, London: Race Equality Unit.

Beresford, P. (1994) *Changing the Culture: Involving Service Users in Social Work Education*, London: CCETSW, Paper 32.3.

Beresford, P. and Croft, S. (1993) *Citizen Involvement: A Practical Guide*, London: Macmillan.

Bignall, T. (2000) *Between Ambition and Achievement: Young Black Disabled People's Views and Experiences of Independence and Independent Living*, London: The Policy Press.

British Association of Social Workers (BASW) (1990) *Managing Care: The Social Work Task*, Birmingham: BASW.

Brown, H. and Smith, H. (eds) (1992) *Normalisation: A Reader for the Nineties*, London: Routledge.

Campbell, J. and Oliver, M. (1996) *Disability Politics: Understanding our Past, Changing our Future*, London: Routledge.

Chappell, A. L. (1997) 'From normalisation to where?' in Barton, L. and Oliver, M. (eds) *Disability Studies: Past, Present and Future*, Leeds: The Disability Press.

Central Council for Education and Training in Social Work (CCETSW) (1974) *Social Work: People with Handicaps Need Better Trained Workers*, London: Central Council for Education and Training in Social Work.

Clarke, M. and Stewart, J. (1992) *Empowerment: A Theme for the 1990s*, Luton: Local Government Management Board.

Dalrymple, J. and Burke, B. (1995) *Anti-oppressive Practice: Social Care and the Law*, Buckingham: Open University Press.

Davis, K. (1981) '23–38 Grove Road: accommodation and care in a community setting', in Brechin, A., Liddiard, P. and Swain, J. (eds) *Handicap in a Social World*, Milton Keynes: Open University Press.

Davis, K. and Mullender, A. (1993) *Ten Turbulent Years: A Review of the Work of the Derbyshire Coalition of Disabled People*, Nottingham: University of Nottingham Centre for Social Action.

Davis, K. and Woodward, J. (1981) 'DIAL UK. Development of the Association of Disablement Information and Advice Services', in Brechin, A., Liddiard, P. and Swain, J. (eds) *Handicap in a Social World*, Milton Keynes: Open University Press.

DeJong, G. (1979) *The Movement for Independent Living: Origins, Ideology and Implications for Disability Research*, East Lansing: Michigan State University Press.

Dominelli, L. (1998) 'Anti-oppressive practice in context', in Adams, R., Dominelli, L. and Payne, M. (eds) *Social Work: Themes, Issues and Critical Debates*, London: Macmillan.

Equal Opportunities Review (EOR) (1996) 'The Disability Discrimination Act 1995', *Equal Opportunities Review*, 65 (January/February).

Fiedler, B. (1988) *Living Options Lottery*, London: King's Fund Centre.

Finkelstein, V. (1980) *Attitudes and Disabled People: Issues for Discussion*, New York: World Rehabilitation Fund.

Finkelstein, V. (1981) 'Disability and the helper/helped relationship', in Brechin, A., Liddiard, P. and Swain, J. (eds) *Handicap in a Social World*, London: Open University/Hodder and Stoughton.

Finkelstein, V. (1991) 'Disability: an administrative challenge', in Oliver, M. (ed.) *Social Work, Disabled People and Disabling Environments*, London: Jessica Kingsley.

Gillespie-Sells, K. and Campbell, J. (1991) *Disability Equality Training*, London: Central Council for Education and Training in Social Work.

Goodley, D. (2000) *Self-Advocacy in the Lives of People with Learning Difficulties*, Buckingham: Open University Press.

Harding, T. and Beresford, P. (eds) (1996) *The Standards We Expect: What Service Users and Carers Want from Social Services Workers*, London: National Institute for Social Work.

Holman, A. and Bewley, C. (1999) *Funding Freedom 2000, People with Learning Difficulties Using Direct Payments*, London: Values Into Action.

Hunt, P. (ed.) (1966) *Stigma: The Experience of Disability*, London: Geoffrey Chapman.

Joseph Rowntree Foundation (JRF) (2000) *Findings: Implementation of the Community Care (Direct Payments) Act*, York: Joseph Rowntree Foundation.

Kestenbaum, A. (1993) *Making Community Care a Reality: The Independent Living Fund 1988–1993*, London: RADAR/DIG.

Kestenbaum, A. (1996) *Independent Living: A Review*, York: Joseph Rowntree Foundation.

Miller, E. J. and Gwynne, G. V. (1972) *A Life Apart*, London: Tavistock.

Morris, J. (1991) *Pride Against Prejudice: Transforming Attitudes to Disability*, London: The Women's Press.

Morris, J. (1993) *Community Care or Independent Living?* York: Joseph Rowntree Foundation.

Morris, J. (1994) *Independent Lives: Community Care and Disabled People*, Basingstoke: Macmillan.

Oliver, M. (1983) *Social Work with Disabled People*, Basingstoke: Macmillan.

Oliver, M. (1990) *The Politics of Disablement*, Basingstoke: Macmillan.

Oliver, M. and Barnes, C. (1998) *Disabled People and Social Policy: From Exclusion to Inclusion*, London: Longman.

Oliver, M. and Sapey, B. (1999) *Social Work with Disabled People*, 2nd edn, Basingstoke: Macmillan.

Payne, J., Brandon, D., Maglajlic, R. and Hawkes, A. (1998) *Direct Payments for Older People*, London: Policy Studies Institute.

Pollitt, C. (1990) *Managerialism and the Public Services*, Oxford: Basil Blackwell.

Priestley, M. (1998) 'Discourse and resistance in care assessment: integrated living and community care', *British Journal of Social Work*, vol. 28, no. 5.

Priestley, M. (1999) *Disability Politics and Community Care*, London: Jessica Kingsley.

Ryan, T. (1999) *Implementing Direct Payments for People with Learning Difficulties*, York: Joseph Rowntree Foundation.

Sapey, B. and Hewitt, N. (1991) 'The changing context of social work practice', in Oliver, M. (ed.) *Social Work, Disabled People and Disabling Environments*, London: Jessica Kingsley.

Shearer, A. (1972) *Our Life*, London: Campaign for Mentally Handicapped People/ Values Into Action.

Shearer, A. (1973) *Listen*, London: Campaign for Mentally Handicapped People/ Values Into Action.

Shennan, G. (1998) 'Are we asking the experts? Practice teachers' use of client views in assessing student competence', *Social Work Education*, vol. 17, no. 4.

Stevens, A. (1991) *Disability Issues*, London: CCETSW.

Topliss, E. and Gould, B. (1981) *A Charter for the Disabled*, Oxford: Blackwell.

Union of the Physically Impaired Against Segregation (UPIAS) (1976) *Fundamental Principles of Disability*, London: Union of the Physically Impaired Against Segregation.

Wilding, P. (1982) *Professional Power and Social Welfare*, London: Routledge and Kegan Paul.

Wilson, A. and Beresford, P. (2000) 'Anti-oppressive practice: emancipation or appropriation?', *British Journal of Social Work*, vol. 30, no. 5.

Wistow, G. (2000) 'Keeping the balance', *Community Care*, 31 August: 18–19.

Wistow, G. and Barnes, M. (1993) 'User involvement in community care: origins, purposes and applications', *Public Administration*, vol. 71 (Autumn), 279–99.

Wolfensberger, W. (1972) *The Principle of Normalisation in Human Services*, Toronto: National Institute on Mental Retardation.

World Health Organisation (WHO) (1980) *International Classification of Impairments, Disabilities and Handicaps*, Geneva: WHO.

Zarb, G. and Nadash, P. (1994) *Cashing in on Independence: Comparing the Costs and Benefits of Cash and Services*, London: Policy Studies Institute.

Chapter 9

Anti-discrimination, work and mental health

Jan Wallcraft

Introduction

Currently in the UK, responsibility for the person considered to be mentally ill lies with the health services, working jointly with local authority Social Services Departments to provide community support. To modify this system, in order to allow the service user more responsibility for, and control of, her/his destiny, is a very considerable task that many lobbying groups and individuals are currently endeavouring to undertake. As Sayce (2000: 129) points out, attempts to achieve a user-led orientation in services, and 'change-alliances' between users and professionals, can be seen in terms of what she terms a 'disability inclusion' model. This is a civil rights based approach which promises, on the one hand, the 'positive' rights of fair opportunities, social adjustments and support and on the other 'negative' rights such as being free of unfair coercion. Of immediate, accessible interest in this respect, and offering the possibility of positive results, are the programmes funded by the Mental Health Foundation (MHF). These programmes offer either a range of vocational activity leading, if desired, to supported or open employment, or advise employers, and providers of education and training, on strategies to improve access for people who have experienced mental health problems.

The MHF is a charity established in 1949 that works in the fields of mental health and of learning disability. Through publications, conferences and events it promotes greater awareness and understanding of mental health problems and learning disabilities and aims to reduce stigma and prejudice. The MHF works closely with mental health service users and offers funding to support community projects and innovative research. In 1997 it established a Mental Health and Employment Programme. Six mental health and employment projects were identified and granted funding to develop their work. These projects all provide examples of how employment discrimination can be countered and I have selected two of them to discuss in particular detail. The first is a 'self-provisioning' 'green' project designed not to have a mental health label attached to it, and which was founded on the basis of a user-'green professional' collaboration. The second is a project supporting people's efforts to get back into paid employment after long absences from the labour market. The project is based in an area of high black and minority unemployment and disadvantage, and it thus addresses multiple forms of oppression.

The relationship between mental health and employment

It has long been recognised that work gives an individual status, a role, a sense of structure to the day and a meaning to life. Perkins and Repper (1996) remind us how when we meet people for the first time, we ask their name, followed by 'what do you do?', meaning 'what is your job' and thus demonstrate that it is the second most important thing we wish to know about an individual. They tell us how, for people whose only identity and relationships depend on their being 'mental patients', work gives an added status and role, particularly if it is outside the mental health system. They stress that, from a psychological point of view, work offers distraction, predictability and enforced activity, all of which lessen the cognitive and emotional problems associated with mental illness. Like Wing (1988) Perkins and Repper have a particular concern with operationalisation of the concept of mental health disability in seeking to open up work and social opportunities for those wishing to embark on a road to employment. Of course it is recognised that both in the projects that I am going to discuss, and more generally, paid employment is not necessarily an aim that is either desired or helpful to users and survivors of so-called 'working age'. It is precisely the way that society so often follows industry in equating a person's worth with a person's productive value that has been so much a subject of criticism in both mental health and the wider area of disability (Chamberlin, 1977; Oliver, 1990; Priestley, 1999). Thus Abberley (1996: 77) comments of the disabled people's movement that, while exclusion from work is a major source of oppression, and while attempts to increase access are not to be denigrated: 'a thoroughgoing materialist analysis of disablement today must recognise that full integration of impaired people in social production can never constitute the future to which we as a movement aspire'. As I hope to show in this chapter, the MHF programme, in nurturing projects that offer access to a wide range of work-related activity and education, from collective 'self-provisioning' to supporting users and their employers in the more conventional areas of job seeking, does very much take account of a critical approach to the utility of paid employment.

Work-related stress is second only to back problems as the biggest occupational health problem in the UK and it is known that being out of work contributes to poor mental health (Buss and Redburn, 1983). Once a mental health crisis has been experienced, work prospects diminish significantly.

Rogers *et al.* in a survey of over 550 people who had used psychiatric services, found that only 11 per cent were in full-time employment. They comment that:

> A number of interrelated factors seem to affect employment after a person has been in hospital. These include: the emotional residue or impact of a mental health crisis; the stigmatising and institutional effects of time spent in the psychiatric system; and discrimination by employers on learning that someone has been given the label of mental illness.
>
> (Rogers *et al.*, 1990: 93)

Barnes (1991), discussing DoE research, lists ten barriers to employment for disabled people: attitudes of work colleagues; medical screening; education; age; experience; appearance; environment of work; transport to and from work; geographical mobility; and shiftworking. In mental health, while many of the other factors are clearly also of importance (Sayce, 2000), experience is a crucial factor. As Barnes notes, the loss of the work habit is of particular importance to employers in terms of the length of a person's unemployment. (It is perhaps worth also noting, in this context, that a number of the barriers to employment for a disabled person can be seen to play a part in the relatively low employment rates of minority ethnic groups, and in the preponderance of women in part time and temporary work.)

In his discussion of the political economy of schizophrenia, Warner (1994) considers how in non-industrial societies that are not based on wage economies, 'unemployment' is a meaningless concept. For someone to assume a productive role is not dependent on their actually seeking employment, or functioning at a consistent level, and they are likely to be 'valued by their community and their level of disability will not be considered absolute' if they are able to make any constructive contribution, since there is 'work' to be done at a number of levels of activity or ability. This may indicate that we should revise our definition of the 'worth' of paid work and be particularly tolerant of including voluntary and part-time work as valid tools in vocational rehabilitation (VR hereafter).

A place to live and a job to go to featured as the main requirements in Rogers *et al.*'s (1990) survey of people experiencing mental distress yet, as the same survey shows unemployment rates among people diagnosed with mental illness are generally high. Indeed, according to the 1997/8 Labour Force survey (cited in Sayce, 2000: 19) only 13 per cent of people with long-term mental health problems are working.

Boy (1987) reviews the literature to test his hypothesis that 'the mental health treatment process is better served when career counselling and development are included' and that 'their inclusion can contribute to the recovery process of clients'. He identifies several advantages resulting from the inclusion of career counselling, including the fact that clients feel they are 'part of the world'. In a similar vein, Ekdawi and Conning (1994), in a review of the literature of several long-term studies, state that work rehabilitation should be seen not only as 'relevant to future employment, but also to the process of social integration'. They emphasise that assuming the role of 'worker' is perceived as a means and a measure of social adjustment and acceptance, not only by the worker him/herself, but by other people in contact with him/her.

They go on to stress the importance of certain components of work rehabilitation, among which are that:

- it should form part of a dedicated, multidisciplinary psychosocial rehabilitation effort which should not be split into specialist parts, such as medical or vocational;
- there should be a continuum of work provision, from a very sheltered environment, through to open employment;
- there should be support for the workers, the employers, the staff and others in contact with the individual to ensure that the rehabilitation effort is sustained.

Warner (1994) cites the findings of Wing (1988), who identified the rehabilitative elements of work as: (a) offering somewhere free from the emotional over-involvement of staying at home, which may exacerbate mental distress; and (b) offering the chance to succeed at something – and thus boost confidence – by achieving a predetermined level of performance which matches ability.

It perhaps should be acknowledged, however, that in industrial societies, where competition is all, ingenuity is needed to provide a non-taxing, stress-free work environment and employers are likely to need the help of VR specialists in identifying how such activity can be provided for people experiencing mental distress. One could assume perhaps, also, that it would be necessary to help them develop and maintain a relationship with the employee that is not only management-oriented but is empathetic and supportive. Floyd et al. (1994: 145) report how participants in a workshop on Counselling and Employee Assistance at Work felt that 'good supervision should include some form of counselling', although the potentially disabling effect of assuming 'counselling' to be a necessity was recognised.

In a personal communication to the author, the late Douglas Bennett (1996a) asserts that it is important to distinguish between occupational therapy and work, citing research of his own from the 1970s. The former, he suggests, is a solitary pursuit, where one has only to satisfy oneself. The latter, by contrast, requires that one is judged by another person, thus opening up the field of interpersonal relationships and consequent contact with 'normality'. Bennett reminds us that work was a component of the care of the psychiatrically disabled at the end of the eighteenth century: Samuel

Tuke, at his Retreat in York, valued work as a means for restraint and felt that if it was physically active it was good for bodily and moral health, presumably on the basis that if people were tired out, not only were they likely to gain eventual physical health but they were less likely to have the energy to be physically disruptive within the asylum.

Moving back to the contemporary context, Bennett (1996a) maintains that work is still 'without doubt a potent tool of great utility and even though, over its years, its importance waxes and wanes, it will remain essential as a social and psychological human function for the psychiatrically disabled, as it is for all of us'. He concludes that occupation for people experiencing mental distress is currently 'lacking in direction' and maintains that while emphasis is being placed on the provision of residential care and daily living skills, 'psychiatrists will once again have to consider the place of occupation in their services'.

In his (1996) paper to the World Association of Psychosocial Rehabilitation Congress, Bond states his guiding principle to be that 'employment in community jobs plays a central role in helping people lead meaningful, satisfying lives'. He goes on to state that such employment, among other things, fulfils a basic human need to be productive and enables a mental health service user to substitute the role of worker for that of 'patient'. In their National Mind survey Rogers et al. (1990) found that most mental health service users rated real work as being second only to housing as their greatest need. Success in finding and keeping a job could influence the direction of other psychiatric rehabilitation services more towards community integration by showing that it is possible to integrate the psychiatric and the 'normal' world. A further justification for finding people real work in real jobs is that it makes economic sense. The user becomes a contributor to the national exchequer, rather than a drain on it. As Herd and Stalker (1996) suggest, the low employment rate of disabled people as a whole is both a poor use of resources and an indication of the fact that workforces mostly do not reflect the diversity of the general population. Thus the role of vocational rehabilitation/resettlement was clearly established as one of both individual and social value.

In the account of the employment projects funded by the MHF which follows, the underlying assumptions are that employment in our society is a social norm, and that VR should always be a component of psychosocial rehabilitation. Whitehead quotes Marie Jahoda, the sociologist, writing in the 1930s who said famously, that work (even if unpaid):

> imposes a time structure on the working day. It enlarges the scope of relations beyond the often emotionally highly charged family relations and those of the immediate neighbourhood: by virtue of the division of labour it demonstrates that the purposes and achievements of the

collectivity transcend those for which the individual can aim: it assigns social status: it clarifies personal identity: it requires regularity.

(Jahoda, quoted in Whitehead, 1994: 42)

Whitehead goes on to comment that work thus represents:

regularity, social and personal contact, daily structure, external validation, personal esteem, normality, the end of the 'sick' role and the chance
to move on to permanent employment.

(Ibid.: 44)

Vocational rehabilitation models

In looking at models of how people might get back into work with a view to guiding its own decisions on funding projects, the MHF considered the framework outlined by David O'Flynn, then Research Psychiatrist at the former Lewisham and Guy's Mental Health NHS Trust (now South London and Maudsley NHS Trust). He describes the VR options currently available to people experiencing mental distress as being of two kinds: (a) job creation; and (b) open employment or education.

Job creation models of VR are outlined by O'Flynn (1998, unpublished) as being of the following kinds:

- Sheltered work: this is widespread, and of an institutional nature. It is funded by health authorities and local authority Social Services depart-ments, or charities, and provides part-time, low-paid work. Historically sheltered work produces poor quality products and takes place in poor work environments. This form of job creation includes industrial therapy units in hospitals (many of which have now been closed) and is often considered exploitative.
- Sheltered Mobile Crew membership: this consists of small teams and offers part-time work, usually in open markets, on similar terms to sheltered work.
- Clubhouse membership: these are community mental health projects, with an emphasis on membership, empowerment and work. The pure model for them originated in the US where the organisations through which they are constituted are independent, and where members live on or attached to the premises. This philosophy has been modified in the UK, where some Clubhouses are directly health and social services owned (also see TEP below).
- Social Enterprise: this is a form of low-paid, part-time job creation VR, with an emphasis on the quality of work and environment, training and power-sharing. They can be described as 'reformed sheltered workshops aspiring to be social firms'.

- Social firms: these are not-for-profit, high street businesses which create jobs for disadvantaged people. They provide full wages and equal opportunities for a mixed able and disabled workforce. A ratio of 'able-bodied' or 'able-minded' workers to disabled of 4:1 is aimed for. The social firm is prominent in Italy and Germany.
- Consumer-run businesses: these are US versions of the social firm, where all the people in the business are consumers of mental health services.

O'Flynn summarises *open employment or education* as one of the following:

- Vocational training: consisting of segregated training in specific skills which leads to job searching in the open labour market.
- Supported education: this comprises support in community, further and higher mainstream education.
- Employment training: this encompasses a variety of approaches adapted from Employment Services, such as job clubs, CV writing and job search skills.
- Transitional employment (TEP): this provides a 3–6 month trial for those seeking employment, in 'entry level' (i.e low-skilled) jobs. TEP aims at eventual 'transition' to the open labour market.
- Supported employment: this model supports people in choosing a job in the open market, in getting such jobs and then in keeping them and developing their careers. It includes reasonable adjustments to the working environment. Good practice will involve the allocation of a Personal Adviser for each jobseeker/worker.

Bennett (1996b) cautions that 'rehabilitation' should be clearly distinguished from 'resettlement'. He defines rehabilitation as 'the business of helping the person to make the best use of his/her remaining abilities to adapt in as normal a social context as possible'. Resettlement, on the other hand 'is the business of resettling the person in the community or in open or sheltered employment. A person may be rehabilitated and remain in hospital but be able to move from a disturbed to a better ward'. Hence, in assessing the support needed by an individual experiencing mental distress, heed should be taken of the simply expressed plea, 'I just want to get a job'.

The MHF projects

Two of the six projects that the MHF funded were 'Ecocraft' in Nottingham and the Haringey Small Jobs and Employment Project. These two projects are the focus of this section and provide an illustration of how the MHF has attempted to fulfil its key aim of countering the stigma and prejudice faced by those who have experienced mental health problems.

The Ecocraft project

The Ecocraft project can perhaps best be described as semi-segregated VR, in terms of the models of open employment discussed by O'Flynn. It was proposed as a part of Ecoworks, a Nottingham based alliance of 'green' professionals and mental health service users. Ecoworks Ltd is a community organisation formed in Nottingham by an alliance between people who have experienced mental distress and a variety of 'green' professionals. It aims to: (a) improve the quality of life for disadvantaged people by supporting them to develop skills and to use these skills to offer each other mutual aid; and (b) to assist people to create a pleasing and sufficiently warm living environment for themselves, to supply each other with affordable food, and warmth for themselves, and to support each other in their care needs. The organisation has turned disused local authority allotments in the city into an ecological project where organic fruit, flowers and vegetables are grown and where alternative building and living styles can be experienced by service users and by the community at large. Under-used buildings have been as it were 'colonised' by the Ecoworks project, which has, in this way promoted its green ethos. It has links with similar 'green' projects in Europe and shares knowledge and good practice with them.

Funding was requested to pay for a worker and associated running costs of a project to develop or enhance the handicraft, wood-working and DIY skills of mental health service users in small home and garden related products, projects and activities. Because DIY activities are traditionally seen as a male preserve, the need was identified in Nottingham for a women-only project where women could have the opportunity to acquire skills and confidence in working with tools and materials.

Ecocraft recognised that mental health service users have to overcome many disadvantages and barriers before they can even consider returning to work. In terms of providing semi-sheltered training as a form of vocational rehabilitation, a primary aim was to ensure that participants had enough support and sustenance to develop confidence in acquiring and applying useful skills.

Drawing the social, work based and environmental aspects of the training together, Ecocraft planned that by providing mental health services users with practical craft and DIY skills they could enable those joining the project to:

- directly improve their own living environment, standard of living and quality of life by production and installation of small products in their own homes and those of others (possibly for payment);
- build their self confidence and sense of self worth;
- improve their possibilities of going on to seek work;

- extend their networks of relationships in the other activities of Eco-works, the networks of the user movement and among 'green activists', thereby improving social integration; and
- widen horizons on issues of design and ecological technology.

A particular feature of the project, and one which set it apart from the others in the programme, was that it was not presented as a mental health service. It was recognised and supported by mainstream mental health services and the majority of its users were people who had been identified as having severe and enduring mental health problems. However, while there was recognition of the need to provide individuals with a project which met their aspirations, and an understanding of their vulnerabilities, there was no formal acknowledgment of their status as mental health service users and a deliberate effort was made not to adopt the normal procedures of admission, review and discharge applied in conventional services. People were regarded as individuals, not as 'cases' and there was a strong emphasis placed on informality within the project. There were no performance standards or goals set for participants. When users had settled into the project and built up trust they were asked what they wanted from the project and this provided information for monitoring outcomes.

The project was innovative in that mental health service users were fully involved with non-mental health workers in developing a project which had the support of the mental health services but no supervision by them. The aims of Ecocraft were to empower people through improving their quality of life through their own efforts. It was believed that such empowerment forms the bedrock from which people can start to rebuild their hopes.

This model of empowerment can be seen as analogous to that of 'alternative development' as outlined by Friedmann (1992), in which the goals of communal activity and mutual support within a local environment are counterposed to those of global production for profit and the needs of the firm. In a wider argument disputing many of the tenets of 'development economics' which enforces dependency on the poor, Friedmann defines empowerment as having three dimensions: social power, political power and psychological power. Social power arises where households acquire skills and resources by means of sharing their knowledge with each other. Political power consists of 'voice', together with the conventional aspect of the right to vote, and to organise to take collective action. Psychological power is described by Friedmann as a 'sense of potency' or self confidence, often deriving from an individual's actions in the spheres of social and political power, through contributing to the wellbeing of the household unit.

Outcomes

Most of the aims of the project were met. It was not possible to move quite as quickly as anticipated and during the period of the MHF funding there was no handyperson work carried out in people's homes. This work will, however, be developed, as the project's medium-term future is assured.

Two craft groups were established. The planned women-only group was formed and led by a trained woman carpenter as project worker. Seven men formed the other group. The women's group, made up of twelve, was extremely successful. Six of the women taking part were long-term users of mental health services, deemed to have been 'institutionalised' and yet, within the security of a woman-led, women-only group, quite prepared to enter new fields. One woman was able to leave formal mental health services and undertake voluntary work and employment training. Many other people tried the activities on offer in the two groups but did not stay. Some of them did, however, benefit from the experiences by establishing networks of new contacts and new interests, including awareness of environment-friendly practices. Administration of the project was carried out by a volunteer who had herself used mental health services.

By employing under-used space in existing workshops, where users were already attending, the Project was relatively cheap to run.

Ecocraft and anti-discrimination

In concluding this discussion of Ecocraft, it is important to note that it addresses a number of forms of discrimination simultaneously. First and foremost, it addresses the traditional segregation of work skills training for people who have mental health problems: no illness-associated entry criteria were set and it was not established exclusively for service users. Second, sexist stereotypes about carpentry as a male preserve have been successfully countered by the development of a strong women-only group. Third, the project has set itself against a number of 'disablist' and pervasive assumptions about the structure of work. It has rejected a number of received opinions: that an individual has to keep to a specified length of time of training, and to timetabled sessions within it, to be able to be worthy of social investment; that a prescribed sequence of augmentation of skills has to be completed and certificated to be of value to the individual or to the wider society; and that formal 'professional' tutoring is required for a skill to be learned. When applied as universal principles of rehabilitation, these are all discriminatory assumptions and it is critical for the service user movement and its allies, as much as the wider society, to challenge them, if social inclusion is to be taken as a serious objective.

MIND in Haringey Small Jobs and Employment Project (SJEP)

Whereas the Nottingham Ecoworks scheme had a focus on craft-based skills which could enhance the ability of service users and others to make their living conditions pleasant and affordable, the Haringey SJEP was funded in order to meet the desire of people unemployed for extended periods of time, subsequent to mental health problems, to get back into employment on the open market. While in Nottingham the model was one of training, in Haringey it was deliberately focused on: (a) supporting employers to identify jobs which would be a suitable match for the range of skills and the range of expectations of job-seekers on the project books; (b) supporting job-seekers through the period of planning for, and adjustment to open employment; and (c) supporting the employers providing work placements, and their employees. Thus the Haringey scheme can be accurately described as a supported employment scheme, falling within the job creation set of VR models outlined by O'Flynn.

It can also very much be seen in terms of Sayce's (2000) discussion of the disability inclusion scenario that was mentioned earlier, where it is the discrimination barriers that society creates for disabled people that are the focus for change, rather than, necessarily, society as such. It is the social distance that is put between those deemed mad and those deemed non-mad that throws up the barriers that are the focus of initiatives like the SJEP.

The project also works innovatively across the MHF's disability fields by drawing on the 'jobcoach' model of support to people with learning disabilities and applying it to mental health. The objective of this model has been both to offer continuing support to people who have found work after recovering from mental health problems, and to assist those seeking work to improve their job search skills.

The context for the project was that there were estimated to be, in 1996, at least 3000 long-term mental health service users in Haringey, of whom more than 75 per cent were unemployed. Haringey is a particularly economically depressed London borough, with a high proportion of young black men in its eastern areas. Following the closure of the local long-stay psychiatric hospital and the establishment of acute services within the borough, a number of people with mental health problems live in community housing, supported by community mental health teams and outreach workers. A survey of 108 service users who were seeking work, carried out for Haringey's Work Tomorrow Conference in October 1994 revealed that:

- 19.8 per cent had administrative, accounting or computing skills;
- 19.1 per cent had professional or technical skills;
- 22.2 per cent had craft skills; and
- 8.6 per cent had skills in caring professions.

While there was sheltered mental health employment provision in Haringey, providing places for a maximum of a hundred clients, most of those questioned were seeking mainstream occupation in the open market. Only the Haringey Small Jobs Project could offer that opportunity.

MIND in Haringey is a registered charity and has offered a range of innovative residential, counselling, advocacy, complementary therapy and day services to people experiencing mental distress for more than twenty years. It has various sources of financial support and gained initial, one year, funding for the SJEP from the North London TEC and the Tottenham Task Force. While this enabled the project to get off the ground with the appointment of an Employment Worker, further funding was needed to consolidate the achievements, strengthen links with employers and continue working with clients who needed longer preparation before starting work. Time was also needed to seek further funding to ensure the viability and continuity of the project.

The project's Employment Worker offers one or more individual assessment sessions to all clients and forms an employment action plan with each. Participants are assessed when they join the service to determine their skills, interests and support needs. An assessment form which provides a holistic profile of the individual is compiled and ongoing vocational guidance meetings and progress reviews are offered. The action plan may include immediate support in finding work, participation in one or more 20-hour Preparation for Work courses, suggestions for further training, continued individual support, or referral to other sources. The Preparation for Work course provides pre-vocational training in jobsearch and social skills to clients who are not yet 'job ready'. In addition to running all these aspects of the SJEP, the Employment Worker also supervises three volunteers, each working for six hours a week, who help in the Preparation for Work courses and the client support group.

Clients in work, or seeking work, are invited to this weekly evening support group which provides a regular space for two hours, for support with placements, training courses and jobsearch. The first hour of the meeting is used for feedback from group members. The second hour is used for more structured training and discussion on topics selected by group members, such as assertiveness, disclosure of mental ill health at work and stress management.

Outcomes

During the two years the project was funded by the MHF it was used by 220 clients of whom thirty-seven moved into employment (paid and unpaid) and twenty-four into training courses. A range of employers, including banks, supermarkets and voluntary organisations, provided work placements. Over 400 guidance sessions and two Preparation for Work courses were offered.

The immediate future of the SJEP is secure. The local Health Authority and a charitable trust have offered funding which should enable the recruitment of an additional Placement Support Worker. There are also plans to locate the project in its own high street, shop front premises. The SJEP has been successful in transferring a learning disabilities supported employment model and tailoring it to the needs of people experiencing mental distress. The traditional learning disabilities jobcoach has been successfully replaced by a personal support programme which takes into account the unique needs of each client. It is important to repeat that ordinary work is recognised as a significant aspiration of many mental health service users.

Other MHF projects

The Glasgow Association for Mental Health applied for funding for an Employment Development Worker to develop Transitional Employment Placements (TEPs) within 'Flourish House' an innovative clubhouse that this user-centred Association had established. The Employment Development Worker's role was to enhance the work environment in the House and identify part-time positions with various employers in Glasgow. These posts would be contracted to the clubhouse and the clubhouse would guarantee that the work involved was performed to a specified level of competence. At the end of the period of MHF funding, 14 clubhouse members, who had an average lengtht of unemployment of eleven years, had completed their placements. Two moved on to full-time employment, one returned to education, three undertook further placements and one joined a mainstream training project.

The Manic Depression Fellowship (MDF) produced a four page 'mental health and work' leaflet helping employers understand the managed-employment approach which they had developed themselves. The focus is on helping employers understand the kinds of difficulty that accompany manic depression and on the kinds of adjustment of work profiles which are most helpful to recovery. Working with 150 of its local support groups, the MDF distributed 5,500 copies of the leaflet.

A service user group called New Horizons Borders on the Scottish/English border set up a Social Enterprise and produced a book of creative work both to raise awareness of people's experiences and to give people meaningful occupation in putting the book together. The project gave employment to one person who coordinated it, but it also gave a lot of confidence building skills to all the other people involved.

A schizophrenia media agency set up a peer-training scheme for mental health service users to gain skills in communicating and presentation for the media. Again this gave employment to the few people who actually worked on the project, so in that way it was a job creation scheme. But just as importantly, by producing training materials and setting up a training programme, it supported users groups to present their own experiences and views to local media in order to endeavour to influence public opinion.

Conclusion: the MHF recovery model

The projects described in this chapter can all be seen to follow a *recovery* model (Sayce, 2000: 132) and this is the kind of anti-discrimination model that is being developed with colleagues at the MHF at the time of writing this chapter. It starts from the premise that recovery is determined by the individual. For some people full-time employment is the only objective that is meaningful and that is going to be, for them, the 'target' outcome. The SJEP-supported open employment route fits such aspirations well, in our view, and can be seen as a demonstration VR project, in areas of high unemployment, where mental health service users face multiple forms of disadvantage. For other people, the objective of working full time may not be one that they and those who care about them feel is consistent with enhanced self esteem or social worth, or that will necessarily increase skill levels or labour marketability; at that point in their lives they may wish to undertake voluntary activities or something that is less stressful, and which would represent for them much more fulfilling outcomes. The Ecocraft project is a demonstration of a way of doing this.

One of the reasons why our approach was criticised by the statutory-type services is probably that there is a pervasive view that: 'if you don't manage to get a job at the end of this process, you've failed'. And that is again setting people up for failure because, of course, it is not easy for anyone who has been unemployed for a long time to obtain work on the open job market.

So really, in broad terms, it is argued that any VR approach has to start by, and then build on, looking at what each person wants out of their life. One can perhaps see this approach as one which conceptualises VR as more like a modular course of study in personal development, with employment modules just some of the non-compulsory options on the course among the many which are on offer to its 'students'. This kind of approach, I suggest, is one that can successfully counter the discriminatory and stereotypical view that people who have had serious mental health problems can function only at the lowest level of vocational expectations, at menial forms of semi-employment.

References

Abberley, P. (1996) 'Work, Utopia and impairment', in Barton, L. (ed.) *Disability and Society: Emerging Issues and Insights*, Harlow: Prentice Hall.

Barnes, C. (1991) *Disabled People in Britain and Discrimination: A Case for Anti-discrimination Legislation*, London: Hurst and Co.

Bennett, D. (1996a) Unpublished letter to the author.

Bennett, D. (1996b) 'Work and occupation for the mentally ill', in Berrios, G. and Freeman, H. (eds) *150 Years of Psychiatry: the Aftermath*, London: Gaskell.

Bond, G. R. and McDonell, E. C. (1991) 'Vocational rehabilitation outcomes for persons with psychiatric disabilities', *Journal of Vocational Rehabilitation*, vol. 1, no. 3.

Bond, G. R. (1996) *Outcomes from Supported Employment Programs for People with Severe Mental Illness*, presentation for WAPR Congress, Rotterdam, The Netherlands, April.

Boy, A. (1987) 'Work and unemployed mental health clients', *Journal of Employment Counselling*, June.

Buss, T. F. and Redburn, F. S. (1983) *Plant Closings and Community Mental Health*, Beverly Hills, CA: Sage.

Chamberlin, J. (1977) *On Our Own*, London: MIND.

Ekdawi, M. Y. and Conning, A. M. (1994) *Psychiatric Rehabilitation*, London: Chapman and Hall.

Floyd, M., Povall, M. and Watson, G. (eds) (1994) *Mental Health at Work*, London: Jessica Kingsley/Rehabilitation Resource Centre.

Friedmann, J. (1992) *Empowerment: The Politics of Alternative Development*, Oxford: Blackwell.

Herd, D. and Stalker, K. (1996) *Involving Disabled People in Services: A Document Describing Good Practice for Planners, Purchasers and Providers*, Edinburgh: Social Work Services Inspectorate for Scotland.

O'Flynn, D. (1998) *Models of Vocational Rehabilitation*, unpublished paper.

Oliver, M. (1990) *The Politics of Disablement*, Basingstoke: Macmillan.

Perkins, R. and Repper, J. (1996) *Working Alongside People with Long-Term Mental Health Problems*, London: Chapman and Hall.

Priestley, M. (1999) *Disability, Politics and Community Care*, London: Jessica Kingsley.

Rogers, A., Pilgrim, D. and Lacey, L. (1990) *People First Survey*, London: MIND.

Sayce, L. (2000) *From Psychiatric Patient to Citizen: Overcoming Discrimination and Social Exclusion*, Basingstoke: Macmillan.

Warner, R. (1994) *Recovery from Schizophrenia*, London: Routledge, pp. 157–8.

Whitehead, A. (1994) 'The transition from work to employment', in Floyd *et al.*, op. cit.

Wing, J. (1988) 'The social context of schizophrenia', *American Journal of Psychiatry*, vol. 135: 1333–9.

Chapter 10

The significance of anti-discriminatory practice

Non-discriminatory discrimination and social advocacy

Dylan Ronald Tomlinson

Introduction

In this chapter I examine the core themes of anti-discriminatory practice that are common to the range of approaches that I outlined in Chapter 1 of this book. I also identify the key distinctions that can be drawn between them, offer an interpretation of the connections between anti-discriminatory practice and occupational interests, and note the significance of work that has been carried out in this field for health and welfare services more generally. At least four types of nomenclature can be noted in relation to the approaches identified in earlier chapters: anti-racist practice; feminist non-oppressive anti-discriminatory practice; anti-discriminatory practice and anti-oppressive practice. In large part, however, it would be fair to say that nomenclature is not seen to be an issue by most of those delineating these practice frameworks.

Core themes

Five common themes can be readily identified: dealing with inequality; taking a non-deterministic stance in relation to people who are discriminated against; countering the power of negative self-images among clients; confronting stereotypes; and situating social work within a context of immanent political and social reaction to 'problem people'.

Dealing with inequality

All approaches are concerned with addressing the kinds of inequality that clients experience which are *outside* the immediate care responsibilities of social workers and which it is difficult for them to do anything about. This is so in several respects. At its most basic, all forms of anti-discriminatory practice emphasise the application of sociological knowledge, in other words that workers should be able to recognise the advantages that most of them possess in terms of class, education, communication skills and the ascribed privileges of affiliation to majority white cultures. This knowledge then enables social workers to both recognise the damaging impact of rejection and derogation of clients who are in socially excluded and marginalised positions, in terms of their adopting a 'subject' powerless, disengaged position *vis-à-vis* their worker, and to conceptualise ways in which egalitarian relationships with clients might be developed. At its simplest level this then means that clients views are solicited and taken seriously in assessment and care planning processes. At another level this involves raising questions about what may be perceived to be discriminatory procedures with superiors, while at its grander levels it means that social workers advocate for their clients by pushing into little examined areas of legal and organisational discretion or that clients' demands for change in the pattern of services are taken up in joint action with them by social workers, or that social workers' facilitate the articulation and development of proposals for change.

Taking a non-deterministic stance in relation to people who are discriminated against

All approaches argue that discrimination is multi-faceted. Most obviously, as Langan and Day's work shows, the analyses all point to the complex nature of attributes which are complementary on the one hand, and contradictory on the other, in terms of people's self definition across social divisions such as ethnicity and gender, or gender and disability. That is to say that while certain advantages generally accrue to, in particular, white males these cannot be readily measured on some kind of scale. Equally it is not possible to easily define how much of that advantage is gainsaid by a white male being disabled. Similarly it does not follow from the sociological identification of the forms of discrimination suffered by black disabled women, that they will necessarily be seen as clients who require a redoubling of professional efforts to address the fact that they suffer disadvantage across three social divisions of ethnicity, gender and disability. This would be both to ignore interaction of these divisions with issues such as class, community solidarity, and diasporic networks and to adopt an ahistorical position in relation to the local experiences of dependence and independence within particular service and organisational contexts.

Countering the power of negative self-images among clients

All versions of anti-discriminatory practice acknowledge that, notwithstanding the necessity of taking a non-deterministic approach, many clients will have so absorbed negative self images that discrimination not only affects them in readily observable discriminatory processes such as those of the systems for application and award of social security benefits, or of social services frameworks for measuring pre-prescribed areas of vulnerability, but also in the less observable ways in which they may find it difficult to articulate needs and demands or to see themselves as deserving of support from others.

Confronting stereotypes

All approaches have a primary concern with stereotypes, with the main forms of stereotypes discussed being: blackness and sexual licence; Asian oppression of women through arranged marriages and dowries; gay and lesbian identity as sex obsessed and morally corrupt; burden and/or uselessness in old age; disability as a deficit to be pitied; and disability also, by way of contrast, characterised as a state of innocence and child like dependency. Each approach to anti-discrimination stresses the importance of social workers confronting the stereotyping that surrounds them in political and popular culture.

Situating social work within a context of immanent political and social reaction to 'problem people'

All accounts have an emphasis on oppression as a social phenomenon that social work not informed by anti-discriminatory practice will tend to reproduce. That is to say that social workers are to avoid victim blaming – thinking that the problem lies with the clients getting themselves into difficulties in the first place – and interpreting the emergency or vulnerability that presents itself in terms of a stigmatised range of problem-containing services on offer, rather than pursuing alternatives by inter-agency work or advocacy or networking within the organisation.

Key distinctions

Dominelli's anti-racist practice provides an approach which sets out an *emphatically political prospectus* for change in social work. It is an approach which makes clear that, for those who accept its importance, there can be no 'soft option' of a comfortable career path following established organisational frameworks for responding to client problems. Social workers are enjoined to 'speak out' where necessary, and because of the likely consequences in doing so, advised, at the same time to develop sound support networks, for emotional and occupational security. They are to question eurocentric and culturally imperialist values, such as those which leave unquestioned the belief that it is a good in itself for children to have both natural parents around in the household as carers and role models, and those which ascribe higher social standing to nuclear families than to other family forms. These values are to be rejected insofar as they are propounded as being in themselves of a superior nature and mobilised to devalue practices in non (Anglo-Saxon) white cultures that are not consistent with them. Social work as a profession is urged to be challenging both within the social services and outside them.

Langan and Day's aims are to present trends in an unfolding redevelopment of practice rather than to set out models of how change should occur. In that sense it would be inaccurate to portray the approach as having singular characteristics with which it can be distinguished from the other elaborations of anti-discriminatory practice. However, the feminist contribution in terms of critical approach to family pathology models of abuse is of note, and, in general terms, the distinctiveness of the approach has been its *highlighting of power relations between men, women and children in families*. Men's roles it is argued, had been often unquestioned in the sense that male authority in familial structures was seen as unremarkable. The feminist contribution to anti-discriminatory practice draws attention to the salience of power in families and households in terms of the gender based cues for assertion and assumption of authority by men and fathers, on the one hand, and for submission and lack of self regard for women, mothers and for female children on the other, which had been underplayed in the dysfunctional family models that preceded the feminist intervention. As Hudson notes in Langan and Day (1992), women's roles as colluders in child abuse have been as much the subject of attention in studies of child sexual abuse as men's perpetrating roles.

Dalrymple and Burke's (1995) characterisation of anti-oppressive practice with clients is analagous to models of liberation struggles in the Second and Third Worlds. In this respect the significant aspects of practice are the exchange of knowledge and skills between all parties; community development, in terms of the building up of relations of trust and mutuality; alternative technologies; political resistance; and social change. An integral part of this process is self liberation, and Dalrymple and Burke's approach, at least in this regard, perhaps offers more encouragement for workers to sustain anti-discriminatory practice and anti-racist practice because its 'personal growth' potential is brought to the fore. Thus this model does not envisage such a necessarily 'hard ride' for those who cleave to this form of approach, as is anticipated by Dominelli. Rather it offers a prospect which is *therapeutic* for all those who are involved. It is this aspect I would suggest that is the key differentiating factor in terms of the model of anti-oppressive practice which Dalrymple and Burke set out.

Thompson's anti-discriminatory practice can perhaps best be described as having *evaluative and reflective objectives* for workers in human services (Thompson, 1997). His approach is one that aims to span professions and disciplines in all areas of 'welfare state' provision. On the whole, he does not locate the main problems of discrimination within the social worker's own cultural make up, or professionalism, though he does of course draw attention to the way in which culture, in particular through ideology, reinforces beliefs about how certain social groups behave, and on the unhelpful assumption of a charitable helping role within professionalism that is problematic in relation to discrimination. But an important point for Thompson is that the wider network of professions in health and welfare, including social work, do actually have access to useful resources to equip them to work in anti-discriminatory ways. One such helpful resource is reflective practice, a model of professional development in which the practitioner builds a framework for responding to client issues jointly with the client, and in the process constantly modifies the techniques that he or she has learned in training and which might be of value. The acts of 'trying out' the techniques to hand leads to the ad hoc development of new approaches, which can best meet the client situations that present themselves. The approach is evaluative in the sense that, as Thompson discusses in relation to age discrimination in Chapter 3 of this volume, it asks for workers to recognise both the way in which the markers of vulnerability, in respect of infirmity and social losses, for example, indicate that to a degree, albeit a degree that one wishes to limit as far as possible, the client's dependence is a fixed aspect of his or her situation, and the degree to which, on the other hand it is of the utmost importance to nurture the client's orientation to a better life in the future, involving self made goals and plans, and to make this an objective of discussion and a measure of agency response.

It should be remembered that these are of course academic approaches to the countering of discrimination, and as Dominelli points out in Chapter 4 of this volume, there were notable differences of view in the profession, during the late 1980s and early 1990s, as to both the desirability and the feasibility of implementing such programmes. One of the intriguing aspects of the integral challenge to dominant moral values, within the white middle class, and to men as dominant within that class, was the question it raised of what form of value system for anti-discriminatory social workers would be developed in their place. A detachment from values would be a contradiction in terms, and value neutrality, as a professional position is of course the very opposite of the social and political engagement that is a central attribute of anti-discriminatory practice. At the same time, to posit that social workers refrain from making positive or negative judgements with regard to an array of value positions inherent in different cultures, would lead to a sense of threat to self and identity, insofar as those latter constructions are accepted as having valid meaning. The injunction to a perpetual acknowledging and throwing into relief of personal values, in order to distinguish the collusions, bases, omissions and other 'unfair' elements within them, in respect of the relationship with the client, could arguably, in the press of business, require stentorian self-discipline and commitment.

A related question is that of what the epistemological basis for the assault on 'dominant values' might be. In other words, what are the knowledge interests and power interests that are implicated in the construction of anti-discriminatory practice, and of the aggregation of people into groups who are judged different; to be the subject of discrimination. If you remove the stigma of social history from your expectations of people as clients they perhaps become something else: people who are ready to freely exchange knowledge and skills; who are ready to grow as individuals; who will share their inmost concerns and allow workers into the private domains of their thoughts and desires; . . . in other words people who are, perhaps, the mirror image of the anti-discriminant practitioner. The expectation of a change in practice, so that it follows empowering and egalitarian principles, will, of itself, be associated with a change in the nature of client responses. This question is addressed more fully in Winston Trew's concluding chapter.

It is clear that, as discussed in Chapter 1, the development of radical social work, and the increasingly important role accorded to social science, mean that belief in a more equal and just society, and that social work has an important part to play in achieving that society, undoubtedly underlie the process by which anti-discriminatory practice has been identified.

It is also the case, I would suggest, that this development can be interpreted as making three claims: first for defensible moral ground; second for a career which has vocational strength – a modest form of social standing or social recognition; and third for occupational stability in the sense of recognition from other occupations and professions for a distinctive set of skills in what can be called, as a convenient form of shorthand, social advocacy. This is a term which includes: care advocacy; client advocacy; citizen advocacy; community advocacy; and intrapersonal and interpersonal advocacy. The profile of this latter claim can be seen in the premium which anti-discriminatory practice places on eliciting the 'authentic' opinions of clients and potential clients, unalloyed by mistrust and the less-than-fulsome communications characterising unequal worker–client relationships, and the full integration into the dialogue between worker and client of an appreciation of the role of cultural and structural inhibitors in shaping the client's situation.

An issue in relation to defensible moral ground is that while social work, in its role of child protection, has been subject to criticism both for its claimed lack of action, tentativeness and lack of decision, it has at the same time, been characterised as over-intervening and bullying (Franklin, cited in Langan and Day, 1992: 139; Philpot, 1999). Other key professions taking part in child protection work appear not to have attracted the same opprobrium.

This set of claims can be seen to be in opposition to the care management, processing and 'product-oriented' social work which is perceived as little able to do more than allot clients to the generic targeted services – family support, domiciliary care, residential care, respite care and so on in as speedy and efficient a way, albeit one that is respectful and listening, as possible.

In relation to the career which has vocational substance, a question that Wilson and Beresford's (2000) critique raises is one of who anti-discriminatory practice is for. They point out that users have not asked for anti-oppressive practice as such, and that it is another possible source of professional aggrandisement in that sense. However this is a curious view when it is considered that one of the most quoted authors in the disability movement has consistently highlighted forms of discrimination within social work (Oliver, 1983, 1991). The logical conclusion of Wilson and Beresford's critique is that no profession should be arrogant enough to claim for itself a set of specialist skills to be able to offer within the health and welfare labour market. Clearly, those espousing anti-discriminatory practice argue that it is a framework which offers the prospect of a redistribution of power, even if, as a consequence, social work becomes a less denigrated, less disadvantaged profession as a by-product of the process. Endemic to that process is the recognition that, in a vocational sense, social workers have agency, valence and privileged insights into the continually shifting patterns of extreme social stress. Some form of desirability of role, some form of social standing, even if this is set out as being in clear distinction to the classic processes of occupational closure which define professions struggling with each other for monopoly of knowledge, may be a legitimate expectation of the redistributive process (Parkin, 1979).

The emphasis on challenge to dominant values, egalitarianism and social advocacy can also be seen to reflect the lack of appeal of what might be termed the 'community protection' function in the late twentieth century – i.e., that function which is based on: limit setting; the enforcement of agreements or contracts between clients and professionals; modelling of behaviour; discipline; and the general deployment of the sanction of authority on behalf of 'society'. To a degree this reflects, within the context of sociology as it has been applied to social work, the profound pessimism of postmodernism, particularly in respect of Foucauldian thought, for which perpetual, unceasing challenge to power is the only respectable and legitimate option, and where even that challenge is problematic insofar as it contains the seeds of desire, from the challengers, to be dominant themselves. Nonetheless, community protection is of course wholly consistent with social advocacy.

Non-discriminatory discrimination

In several significant senses, anti-discriminatory practice in health and welfare services is a contradiction in terms. First, the organisation of British and other European societies, reinforced by the trading objectives of the EU (Deacon, 2000: 80–1), is such as to support and reward entrepreneurial activity, the creation of wealth through industry and through the exchange of goods and services. Social solidarity is secondary to and is dependent on the success of trade. Since trade involves the accumulation and concentration of profits, its outcome is always one which is: flaunted as a matter of principle; discriminatory against the workers from whose employment profits are derived; and belittling to those who are unsuccessful in or who do not have the means of access to, the entrepreneurial field. The necessity for the state to provide compensatory services for the marginalised and excluded is a corollary of such processes. More importantly the provision of such services is intended as, famously in respect of National Assistance in the Beveridge Report (1942), a merely temporary expedient, and to be directed at sustaining those who experience hard times only until they can sell their labour for a sufficiently high price, within the politically and culturally sanctioned framework of the free market, to achieve a status above the level of compensatory services.

Second, discrimination takes place through the rationing of services, means testing, and the application of charging policies. Health and social services have always been subject to the constraints of national economic conditions and, even in left-of-centre social democracies, the principle of maintaining high levels of taxation for welfare is a well contested one (George, 1998). Services are in all instances organised on the basis of discrimination between those judged to be in need of assistance and those judged not to be in need of assistance, even if these groups are no longer conceptualised as, respectively, the deserving and the undeserving (Sanderson, 2000). It is a salient political concern within liberalism that the receipt of support from the state should not be sufficiently attractive that it detracts from the individual's pursuit of work, and through it the means of lifelong self-support and planning for the contingencies of indigence and dependence.

Third, the well-documented 'surveillance' function (Rodger, 1996) of health and social services illustrates the degree to which they discriminate in terms of discipline. The practice distinctions that are drawn in terms of what is acceptable and what is questionable in clients' own care-giving, within the specialisms of health visiting, social work, probation, and youth work are reinforced, as several contributors to this volume point out, by the ideological policing that takes place in the media. The media regularly mobilise popular feelings and perceptions against, for instance: benefit recipients as scroungers living on hand-outs; people coming into the UK from the Indian sub-continent as maintaining separate cultures and languages to undermine the hypothesised English culture and the English language; and lesbian and gays promoting lifestyles that are confusing and distressing for children having to grow up in lesbian and gay households. These biases require constant vigilance, on the part of social workers if they are to be countered and rejected within the social work imagination. However, the effects of the mobilisation of bias cannot be prevented entirely from having a discriminatory impact as they frequently lead to government circulars pandering to public opinion in, for example, giving rulings and placing limitations on professional and organisational discretion in areas such as those concerning refugees and asylum seekers, and people undergoing mental health crises.

Fourth, the decision making that is involved in practice inevitably draws on frameworks which define client behaviour as being within or not within tolerable margins. The concept of so-called good enough parenting, for example, indicates how care giving by clients can be judged to contain within it sufficiently nurturing, tolerable levels of anger, contempt for, or disaffection from those cared for, in terms of a borderline with abusive care. Such discrimination is clearly both, on the one hand, incorrigibly subjective and on the other, affirming of the preferred cultural values of the society, about emotional and physical violence, about the significations of 'caring about', about ability and vulnerability, albeit that such discrimination is constantly changing and adapting to circumstance.

Fifth, the doubts within and outside medicine about the extent to which it can be regarded as health advancing (Illich, 1975; Mckeown, 1976) both carry over into social work in those areas that are closely related to medicine, such as disability, and have parallels within those areas that are less closely related (Thompson-Cooper, 2001). The recourse to social services may be argued to sap the autonomic potential of networks of community succour and protection: institutionalisation has been widely noted as marked by processes of loss of volition and independence. Equally, social work has been noted to have a thin evidence base in terms of proven effectiveness (Editors, 1998) and it may be plausibly asserted to a degree, that social services are iatrogenic in nature.

These inherent contradictions suggest that it would be perhaps more accurate to describe anti-discriminatory practice as anti-discriminatory discrimination or non-discriminatory discrimination. In other words, that it embodies an *aspiration* to counter discrimination in all professional actions but an acknowledgment that in many instances the offering of services and legitimation of unwanted interventions will in itself reinforce social discrimination.

The significance of anti-discriminatory practice for health and welfare

What I hope to have drawn attention to in this discussion is that it is the *process* of anti-discriminatory practice, rather than its outcome, that is of the keenest interest in respect of health and welfare more widely. A hallmark of that process is the strength of application of social science to practice considerations.

In this respect, probably the most significant aspect of anti-discriminatory practice in relation to health and welfare services more widely, is its intrinsic social monitoring and evaluation function. This embodies the requirement for continual work-based study and reappraisal of culture, in all its aspects; of the shifting nature of identity and the changing boundaries between social groups; and the ever emergent representation of different needs and demands within and between such groups. In being distinctive of anti-discriminatory practice it is this kind of work that constitutes, as it is reported, discussed and disseminated, a highly significant resource for other agencies to 'tap' into.

A second important aspect for the wider service context is that of social advocacy as it has been outlined above. Such advocacy provides rich opportunities for joint work between professions, and between professions and user/carer organisations, especially with regard to the scope for a response to need which acknowledges the multifaceted nature of discrimination, implicating the consideration of a wide range of areas of care and support, often outside the compass of the NHS and social services, if the service user's construction of their situation is to be taken seriously.

Third, social advocacy, in so far as social work premised on anti-discriminatory practice tends to lead to specialism within it, indicates the scope for the development of inter-professional and inter-agency educational and training resources, particularly those which may connect professional and service user agencies. Rather than the 'purist research' which is under-taken by specialist bodies, small to medium scale practitioner–service user evaluations, audit and exploratory studies of unfolding patterns of discrimination and responses to them, would provide a strong foundation for social advocacy. Such evaluative studies also highlight in addition the importance of research being contracted from users and carers organisations as well as for users and carers organisations to be supported to initiate their own analyses and investigations. The intrinsic nature of monitoring and evaluation processes suggests, at the same time, that the field of anti-discriminatory practice, with all its contradictions, and under whatever nomenclature turns out to be preferred in the future, can provide significant staff development opportunities.

References

Beveridge, W. (1942) *Social Insurance and Allied Services*, London: HMSO.

Deacon, B. (1997) *Global Social Policy: International Organisations and the Future of Welfare*, London: Sage.

Dalrymple, J. and Burke, B. (1995) *Anti-Oppresive Practice: Social Care and the Law*, Buckingham: Open University Press.

Editors, (1998) 'What makes you think it will work? – A conversation with Brian Sheldon about evidence-based social services', *Management Issues in Social Care*, vol. 5, no. 1.

George, V. (1998) 'Political ideology, globalisation and welfare futures in Europe', *Journal of Social Policy*, vol. 27, no. 1.

Illich, I. (1975) *Medical Nemesis: The Expropriation of Health*, London: Calder and Boyars.

Langan, M. and Day, L. (eds) (1992) *Women, Oppression and Social Work*, London: Routledge.

McKeown, T. (1976) *The Role of Medicine: Dream, Mirage or Nemesis?* Oxford: Nuffield Provincial Hospitals Trust.

Oliver, M. (1983) *Social Work with Disabled People*, London: Macmillan.

Oliver, M. (ed.) (1991) *Social Work, Disabled People and Disabling Environments*, London: Jessica Kingsley.

Parkin, F. (1979) *Marxism and Class Theory: A Bourgeois Critique*, London: Tavistock.

Philpot, T. (ed.) (1999) *Political Correctness and Social Work*, London: IEA Health and Welfare Unit.

Rodger, J. J. (1996) *Family Life and Social Control: A Sociological Perspective*, Basingstoke: Macmillan.

Sanderson, I. (2000) 'Access to services', in Percy-Smith, J. (ed.) *Policy Responses to Social Exclusion: Towards Inclusion?* Buckingham: Open University Press.

Thompson, N. (1997) *Anti-Discrimination Practice*, Basingstoke: Macmillan.

Thompson-Cooper, I. K. (2001) *Child Welfare Professionals and Incest Families: A Difficult Encounter*, Aldershot: Ashgate.

Wilson, A. and Beresford, P. (2000) 'Anti-oppressive practice: emancipation or appropriation?', *British Journal of Social Work*, vol. 30, no. 5.

Chapter 11

Making a difference? From anti-racist to anti-oppressive practice in social work education

Winston Trew

Introduction

The last two decades of the twentieth century have witnessed the rise and fall of anti-racism in social work education and training, following closely on its demise in local politics (Gordon, 1991; Gilroy, 1990). It is ironic that having once been hailed as a more radical policy and strategy over 'racism awareness training' (RAT) (Sivanandan, 1985; Gurnah, 1985; Stubbs, 1985), and from promising solutions to problems of service relevance and service delivery to those discriminated on grounds of 'race' (Dominelli, 1999), anti-racism is now regarded as a problem in itself. Hostile media coverage of 'same-race' placements policy and practice in social work over 1993 and 1994 presented anti-racism as part of an 'Orwellian nightmare' and as a prime example of 'political correctness out of control' (see Jones, 1993, for a critical summary of the media coverage; Pinker, 1993, for an opposing view). For some practitioners and academics, it was seen as part of a campaign of destabilisation by the press and the so-called New Right (Jones, 1993; Singh, 1994). Kirton (1995) suggests that this representation of 'same-race' placements policy and practice proved a watershed in anti-racism in social work, marking the limits of tolerance for anti-racist policy in its public services role.

Even though much of the most recent and vocal criticisms of anti-racism have come from the media and the (not so) New Right, criticisms have none-theless come from black practitioners (Ahmed, 1990) and academics (Gilroy, 1990; Trew, 1992; Singh, 1996; Bonnett, 1993). Ahmed and Singh criticise anti-racism for lacking a black perspective, while Gilroy observes that anti-racism reduces the complexity of black life to just fighting racism. Those working from a black perspective (Ahmed, 1990; Singh, 1996) go on to criticise (mainstream) anti-racism for working from an implicitly 'white perspective', evidenced by its objectification and pathologisation of black populations and cultures as 'Other' (Stubbs, 1985; Rattansi, 1994; Singh, 1996), as opposed to providing a deconstruction of 'Englishness' and 'whiteness' (Rattansi, 1994; Bonnett, 1993, 2000).

While there are those who continue to see anti-racism as relevant to the preparation of the social worker for the future (Singh, 1994), anti-racism has effectively been replaced by anti-oppressive theory and practice on social work teaching programmes (see for instance Braye and Preston-Shoot, 1996; Macey and Moxon, 1996; Dalrymple and Burke, 1995; Adams *et al.*, 1990). Why has anti-oppressive practice become so attractive and so popular among social work educationalists, and what are its advantages over the anti-racism it has come to replace? How does the elevation of 'difference' enable a better insight into the complex dynamics of oppression and empowerment, and the construction of the subject? These are the questions with which this chapter is concerned.

In examining the theoretical underpinnings of anti-oppressive practice, my principal aims are to try to specify how anti-oppressive theory has constructed its vocabulary and how it has defined its field of operation, together with appropriate areas for intervention. One of the claims by those who elaborated anti-racist strategies was that they represented a more radical form of oppositional practice than the multi-culturalism which they had displaced. However, it can be argued that anti-racism may be seen to have incorporated multi-culturalism rather than to have replaced it. Anti-oppressive practice makes a similar claim (i.e. that it is more radical), in relation to anti-racism. So it is therefore necessary to examine this claim on a theoretical level and look at the strategic implications of the types of change this approach advocates.

I begin with an evaluation of anti-oppressive theory and practice within the context of its own claims, then go on to offer a critique of two of its core concepts: 'difference' and 'power', arguing that in their conceptualisation and operationalisation they are open to some of the same charges of theoretical and strategic inadequacy as those that were levelled at anti-racism. I suggest that the emergence of anti-oppressive theory and practice in social work education and the (truth) claims it now makes on the issues of 'difference', 'identity', 'power' and 'empowerment' have come to be located precisely in the spaces where anti-racism has encountered problems in sustaining its own truth claims. The chapter concludes with a discussion of the wider context of power, beyond social work, which any strategy that follows on from anti-racism has to address.

Defining anti-oppressive theory and practice

Anti-oppressive theory and practice distinguishes itself from anti-discriminatory practice and anti-racism in the following ways. According to Dalrymple and Burke (1995: 3) 'anti-oppressive practice is about minimising the power differences in society'. Following Phillipson (1992), they go on to state that this form of practice 'works with a model of empowerment and liberation that requires a fundamental rethinking of values, institutions and relationships' (ibid.). Anti-discriminatory practice, in contradistinction, has the limited aim of working within the existing 'rights' based legislative framework to challenge unfair treatment on ground of 'race', gender and disability, through devices such as the Sex Discrimination Act (1975), the Race Relations Act (1976) and the Disability Discrimination Act (1996). While adherents of anti-discriminatory practice are often critical of the political arrangements which support this framework, Dalrymple and Burke (1995) suggest that they generally accept its constraints. A limitation of anti-discriminatory practice, in this respect, in terms of the critical regard in which it is held by anti-oppressive practitioners, is that it does not advocate challenge to power differentials and structural inequalities between groups and individuals as its *primary* mode of operation. Anti-oppressive practice, then, by contrast means recognising power imbalances and working towards the promotion of change to redress the balance of power.

At a theoretical and strategic level, anti-oppressive practice claims to overcome some of the limitations of anti-racism in that: (1) it flattens out any notion of a 'hierarchy of oppression', with the centralisation of a single, unifying variable, 'difference'; and (2) it moves beyond the exclusivity of the category 'black' offered by anti-racism, by recognising the existence of multiple forms of oppressions and identities in society (Dalrymple and Burke, 1995; Macey and Moxon, 1996; Preston-Shoot, 1995). As explained by Macey and Moxon:

> the shift from anti-racist to anti-oppressive social work education is radical rather than reactionary. It moves from the narrow, exclusive focus on racial oppression to a broader, more inclusive understanding of the links between various forms and expressions of oppression.
>
> (Macey and Moxon, 1996: 309)

Singh (1996: 42) is more cautious about these claims since anti-oppressive practice will have to overcome that which had defeated anti-racism over the years: the hegemony of the white, middle-class, male, non-disabled and heterosexual 'mythical norm' in defining normality, and the denigration of everything that stands outside its construct. He thinks that 'anti-oppressive practice will not be able to challenge this state of affairs unless there is some concrete means of constructing, an alternative state of consciousness based on a celebration of difference'. He adds that, crucially:

> If oppression operates to deny the legitimacy to one's identity and difference, then anti-oppressive practice must be doing the opposite; that is validating and nurturing difference.
>
> (Singh, 1996: 42)

In view of the problems he foresees with the development of anti-oppressive practice Singh calls for an expansion of anti-racism to include 'black perspectives' rather than an abandonment of it. However, whereas Singh sees oppression as characterised by the *denial* of difference, Preston-Shoot's definition of oppression focuses on the *exploitation* of difference:

> At the root of oppression is difference, whether age, sexuality, ethnicity, gender, class, financial resources or behaviour. Dominant groups may exploit these differences, stigmatise them, or control them. Those regarded as different are ignored, devalued, blamed, dehumanised, with their differences used to 'justify' the reaction.
>
> (Preston-Shoot, 1995: 15)

The axis on which the various forms of oppression turn in anti-oppressive theory is 'difference': how dominant groups use the differences between people as causal factors in their marginalisation, exclusion, persecution and exploitation. In the work of Dalrymple and Burke the concept of difference comes to occupy a central place in anti-oppressive theory. Speaking about the experiences of women, they explain that:

> Black women are treated differently from white women, lesbians are treated differently from heterosexual women, disabled women are viewed differently from able-bodied women, older women are viewed differently from younger women. We live in a society characterised by 'difference', but these differences are not viewed positively. Differences are used to exclude rather than include. This is because relationships in society are the result of the exercise of power on individual, interpersonal and institutional levels.
>
> (Dalrymple and Burke, 1995: 8)

I want to raise a number of problems with this formulation of difference and its assumed role in oppression and liberation as conceptualised by Singh, Preston-Shoot and Dalrymple and Burke. The problems I raise are not theirs exclusively, but part of a common language and set of practice-concepts currently dominant in what may be termed broadly as 'counter-hegemonic' practices within social work education. For example, the validating body of the social work profession, CCETSW requires teaching institutions that offer Diploma programmes to provide evidence that their training works to counter discrimination by, for example, students developing an 'understanding of concepts such as normality and difference', among other anti-discrimination evidence indicators (CCETSW, 1995). Here difference is presented as both the *basis* of the problem and its *resolution*. What seems to be required is a reversal of power relations and a valuing of 'difference'. Anti-oppressive practice therefore seems to come with a 'theory' of how the problem is constructed and with a ready-made strategy for its resolution.

The dominance of the discourse of difference and its diffusion in the political culture of society can be highlighted by noting its use in 1999 by a Labour MP, who declared that 'we are all different' in response to media questioning about his sexuality in the wake of his sudden and controversial resignation as a Minister (*The Observer* 1 November 1999). The implication was that his *difference* was being used to discriminate against him, and that this *difference* ought to be respected and not be used as a device or vehicle for persecution. Immediate questions that are raised here are these: 'from what or from whom are all these groups that are oppressed for being "different", actually different?' If every one is equally different, then that begs the further question, 'where is the place that this power of definition is being applied from against these groups?' If these groups all constitute various forms of the 'Other', what then, is the identity of the 'Self', the nature of the 'Same' or location of the 'Centre'? In short, who or what observes all these 'differences' as different? To whom does the 'gaze' belong? What is it that Sees but is not Seen?

The problem with 'difference'

I have three main concerns with the above formulation of 'difference' as the axis of oppression/liberation, each of which is explored in turn below:

1   There is a failure to interrogate the concept and application of 'difference' theoretically. The use of the concept appears on the one hand to be rooted primarily in biological discourses and second in social relations, in that 'differences' seem to exist *prior* to the application of the power to denigrate, 'deny and oppress'. More problematical, the 'differences' claimed for authentication and celebration appear to coincide with what Cocks (1989) calls the 'brute fashionings' of 'race' and gender typologies and boundaries established by previous forms of racism, and other hegemonic discourse. In other words, crude typologies of racial difference seem to have been replaced by ethnic difference.

2   There is a tendency to see power as one-dimensional – as applied from above, on to pre-existing differences below. Though anti-oppressive practice implies an understanding of the interpersonal nature of power relations, it seems to operate within a reductionist model of power, and fails to analyse power not just as centralised in institutions and social structures but as dispersed throughout society in a web of power–knowledge relations involving individual subjects.

3   There is a failure in the literature to deconstruct the hegemony of the 'white mythical norm' – the absent centre, which, I suggest, is the site and place from where all these differences are being observed, constructed

and signified. 'Difference' is always 'distance' from a point of reference of privileged 'invisibility' – a site which needs to be interrogated (Singh, 1996; Rattansi, 1996; Bonnett, 1993).

What is difference?

Discourses on difference rely on 'differences' which are understood primarily in the context of discourses on bodily or biological difference, to which the categories of gender and 'race' belong (Schilling, 1993). In this respect Connell, cited in Schilling (1993: 108) posits that the major inequalities within society are based on differences *without permanent (or absolute) foundation in the body*. Far from being the expression of natural difference exclusive gender identities are based on the suppression of gender similarities and an *exaggeration of differences*. This has been the result of the negation or suppression of biology in social theory (Schilling, 1993: 108–9). Connell terms this contradiction between the 'social processes of categorisation and the bodily bases' on which these rest, 'the negation of biology'. However, by negation he does not suggest 'the complete negation of biology, but rather its distortion'.

Hegemonic discourses therefore distort the role of biology in the construction of social identities so that the 'distorted fashioning' of bodily forms, their imagery and significance comes to act as a seemingly pre-social and pre-discursive site for individual identity and therefore difference. Cocks (1989: 20) refers to these embodiments as 'brute fashionings' because they take the form of rudimentary and naively given differences which are then offered as a basis for our social identity and self-recognised difference from one another. So, for example, though women and men differ enormously in their height, weight, strength, endurance, and the distribution of these features overlaps between the sexes, the production of men and women as separate and unequal categories operates by converting the average or relative differences into absolute differences (Schilling, 1993: 109) so that an individual from that group can be assumed to embody all of the characteristics which define or 'fashion' that group.

For Liff and Wajcman (1996) difference is always constructed in relation to the category of other. Drawing on poststructuralist feminist theory (Weedon, 1987; Fuss, 1989), they propose that 'we understand male and female characteristics in relation to each other rather than as independent categories. More importantly, the construction of "woman as different" embodies a notion of "different from male"' (Liff and Wajcman, 1996: 87). This is coupled with a rather one-dimensional view and understanding of how power operates, in that it is assumed that power is exercised from above and acts negatively on supposed self-evident differences, rather than that hegemonic power is actively involved in the production and reproduction of gender difference. That is to say that marked differences between men and women, and between black and white people (as social and cultural categories) are actually constructed in the political process of definition by those wielding various forms of power. Thus Soja and Hooper argue that:

> Hegemonic power does not simply manipulate naively given differences between individuals and social groups, it actively *produces and repro-duces* difference as a key strategy to create and maintain modes of social and spatial divisions that are advantageous to its continued empowerment.
>
> (Soja and Hooper, 1993: 184–5, emphasis added)

The articulation of women's subordination therefore occurs within a 'phallo-centric' discourse, where 'the presentation of (difference as) a single binary division between men and women both polarises the difference between them and exaggerates the homogeneity of each category' (Liff and Wajcman, 1996: 87). Turning to anti-racist theorising, it can be argued that it is not that black people are racially or culturally different, but that black subjects are used in racial discourse to denote racial difference in essentialist and naturalised terms (Trew, 1992; Liff and Wajcman, 1996). I propose therefore that we understand discourse as constituting differences rather than just reflecting them negatively, as assumed in the frameworks of anti-oppressive theory and practice discussed above.

Undoing the masculine, heterosexual, able-bodied, mythical 'white norm'

I want to elaborate on Liff and Wajcman's (1996) point about the gendered (and racialised) production of difference, and how phallocentric discourses signify women as different from men; as identifiable by an absence of male characteristics in similar ways to those in which black people are variously constructed as identifiable by an absence of white characteristics. Phallo-centrism is a term used by feminists to describe the 'patriarchal symbolic order'. It arises from critiques and deconstructions of Freud's psychoanalysis in which women were signified as the sexual other of men because they had no penis – a defining male characteristic. The phallus was elevated to stand as a sign for, and representative of, the patriarchal symbolic order in which men are dominant, and their dominance seen as a 'law of nature' (Grosz, 1990). Phallocentrism therefore refers not only to the symbolic centralisation of the male organ, 'but to the continuing subversion of women's autonomy in the norms, ideals and models devised by men' (Grosz, 1990: 174). This read-ing coincides with what Singh (1996) referred to as the 'white male mythical norm' and the 'absent centre' of post-structuralism.

The point I want to make is that it is phallocentrism that signifies white women as different from white men, sexually, physically and psychologically.

It does not signify them as different from black, heterosexual women or lesbians: their primary site of difference is difference from men on the authority of the phallus, not from other women. This is an important point. But it is necessary to state here that I am not suggesting that the various differences between the subordinate groups represented in the quotation from Dalrymple and Burke (p. 163) are illusions or fictions. My point is rather that I am suggesting, following Lacan (cited in Game, 1991: 74), that the perception of these differences by the subject groups, in the ways that they regard each other, and themselves, 'is not a seen gaze but a gaze *imagined* . . . [by them] . . . in the field of the Other' (emphasis added). That is to say that difference stems from a particular 'looking' which needs to be interrogated.

This 'gaze', that sees difference in the 'field of the Other', may be described as the internalised gaze of the Self mediating the 'looking' of the different – the 'Other' – at themselves in the form of 'truth claims'. These 'truth claims' are dispersed throughout society by way of a range of normalising discourses through which we take up our classed, gendered, sexed and racially embodied subject positions within a structured symbolic order.

Humphries (1997) helpfully connects discourse, power and the construction of 'reality' in the form of 'truth claims' as follows:

> Discourse is a form of social practice which does not just have the effect of representing, but of signifying the world, constructing it in meaning. It constitutes social subjects, social relations and systems of knowledge and the study of discourse focuses on its constitutive ideological effects. It refers to a 'set of meanings, metaphors, representations, images, stories, statements' . . . that in some way together produce a particular version of events. . . . Foucault identified discourse as historically variable ways of specifying knowledge and truth – what it is *possible* to speak at a given moment. Discourses produce truths and 'we cannot exercise power except through the production of truth'.
>
> (Humphries, 1997: 642, emphasis added)

The knowledges we use to understand 'self' and 'other' (who I am/am not) are simultaneously mediated by multiple discourses operating at the linguistic, symbolic, cultural and political-economic levels of society. Subjects become subjects by both accommodating and resisting discourse, by playing with, rejecting and manipulating meaning. Thus, according to Fox:

> Personal identities emerge not as a prior and privileged ontology, but in a 'battlefield', in which difference and opposition are means by which identity, and the boundaries of others become discernible.
>
> (Fox, 1998: 426)

I have so far identified 'power' and 'difference' as key concepts in anti-oppressive theory and practice. I have suggested that because of the way that the concept of difference is applied in everyday discourse as well as in social work literature, we are compelled to see others and understand ourselves in terms of the differences given – which I have argued are actually the effects of the application of power. Rather, analysis should focus attention on the discourse and power relations that are involved in the creation and mobilisation of difference concepts. In other words, it is necessary to locate the situations in which difference concepts are mobilised and to find out how those situations are structured in relation to particular discourses.

Looking again at power and its application in the production of bodily difference(s), and their 'subject positions' in discourse, Kerfoot and Knights apply Foucault's analysis of power, knowledge and discourse in the production of gender and sexual identity, to argue that:

> power is the effect of strategies and mechanisms embedded in social practices which are themselves the consequences of the application of the operations of previous power/knowledge relations and apparatuses. This is to suggest that power has a history, albeit discontinuous. In its exercise however, power is targeted upon bodies and social relations in such ways as to discipline individuals and regulate populations. Foucault's work on discipline identifies hierarchical surveillance, normalising procedures and the 'examination' as the three most dominant strategies or instruments of power in modern society. The power of each strategy lies in their effect not just in constraining subjects through external observation, segregation and judgment of populations, *but also in producing a subjectivity that generates its own self-discipline internally, within people. In other words, the concern is how subjectivity is produced – how individuals come to recognise themselves as subjects and, in turn, are recognised by others.*
>
> (Kerfoot and Knights, 1994: 82–3, emphasis added)

What is suggested by Kerfoot and Knights is that subjects are not only fashioned by 'external' disciplinary and regulating institutions (family, education and employment), and normalising discourses such as 'race', gender, sexuality and class, but that subjects also fashion and regulate themselves by an 'internalisation' and 'manipulation' of these discourses and their 'truth claims'. This fashioning takes place within specific historical and political conditions, within pre-given social, cultural and political constraints, and within prevailing 'regimes of truth'. 'Regimes of truth' are the signifying effects of power/knowledge relations that establish which knowledge(s) become possible or admissible as 'truth'. Discourse, as has been discussed, 'refers both to the historical sets of practices which limit human actions and what may be thought, *and* to the theoretical concepts which account for the fact that human beings actually do act and think in line with these regimes of truth' (Fox, 1998: 426, original emphasis). It is through resistance and accommodation, internalisation and objectification that meaning, self-understanding (subjectivity), and therefore identity, is produced. Thus, the individual is 'continually making and remaking his or her identity through a process of coming to terms with personal experiences of the world and, simultaneously, projecting conceptions of that experience back onto the world. The "subject" plays with meaning in order to gain understanding.' Identity, and therefore difference, is not something fixed, innate or natural, but discursively produced and can therefore change according to the situation or context. The possibility of (any) change relies on an understanding of the difference between what one is *identified as*, and what one *identifies with*. It indicates that one is born into a given set of circumstances, and within the limits of the 'regimes of truth' that govern those locations. Those localised truths also govern the types of discursive practices and technologies of the self a particular subject can access or manipulate to bring about change. Foucault sums up this duality of power and 'subjecthood' as follows:

> This form of power applies itself to everyday life which categorises the individual, marks him by his own individuality, attaches him to his own identity, imposes a law of truth on him which he must recognize and which others have to recognize in him. It is a form of power which makes individuals subjects. There are two meanings to the word subject; subject to someone else by control and dependence, and tied to his own identity by a conscience or self-knowledge. Both meanings suggest a form of power which subjugates and makes subject to.
>
> (Foucault, 1982: 212)

Though Foucault speaks in the masculine, the text serves to show that the normalising and hegemonic discourses on gender, racial and sexual identity and difference become the spaces in which, as subjects, we are placed. This placing tends to limit individuality to a 'set of very specific patterns', such as 'race', gender, class, and sexuality. We both recognise ourselves by these patterns and are recognised by them by others.

I have taken this approach to power, difference and identity to provide a critique of anti-oppressive practice at the theoretical level, and, as I suggested at the beginning of this chapter, to examine how far anti-oppressive practice can, in the light of such a critique, realistically offer insights into the dynamics of oppression, empowerment and the construction of the subject. Given that anti-oppressive practice is interested in the empowerment of oppressed and marginalised subjects, theoretically there is a tendency to conceptualise power as 'negative', thus making the subject appear passive and with little if any agency. Moreover, in critiquing the assumption in anti-oppressive theory that identity and difference are obvious, self-existent traits, and a reflection of some biological essence, I have argued to the contrary that biological difference is just one variable in the making and remaking of gender identity.

Looking at the gaze

Returning to the subject of the 'gaze', and the relationships between the 'gaze', regimes of truth, self and 'other', I have already suggested that the perception and markers of say 'race' and gender difference are the effects of a 'mediated seeing', one filtered through the prism of power/knowledge relations. I want to pursue this further. I suggested above that the perception of difference by subjects of one another is not a 'seen gaze' but one 'imagined' by them in the 'field of the other'. Sheshgadri-Crooks (2000: 67), describes the 'gaze' as that which 'situates' the subject as always, already 'given to be seen'. The subject is, above all, characterised by 'its looked-at-ness', which, she suggests, indicates the 'pre-existence of the gaze', as the subject sees from only one point but is seen from many sides. 'Thus the gaze locates the subject as a screen, or a receptacle for the gaze. It makes the subject visible. . . .'

Speaking of racial difference, Sheshgadri-Crooks suggests that it is the 'symbolic order of difference' that orders seeing, rather than the reverse. This is because 'We believe in the factuality of difference in order to see it . . .' (p. 5). What she calls the 'master signifier' – whiteness – establishes 'a structure of relations, a signifying chain that through a process of inclusions and exclusions constitutes a pattern for organising human differences. This chain provides subjects with certain symbolic positions such as "black", "white", "Asian", etc., in relation to the master signifier' (p. 4). In short, though seeing is both structured and ordered, this seeing takes place within the angle of a gaze patterned and ordered by a 'master signifier', a structure, which according to Derrida (cited in Davies and Schleiffer, 1991: 160) 'structures yet itself escapes structurality'. It is what I referred to above as that which 'sees but is itself not seen', that names but has no name.

The only apparatus which subjects have available for perceiving themselves is that of the order provided by the 'gaze'. Taking the subjects identified by Dalrymple and Burke (1995) and Preston-Shoot (1995), seeing through the order of the 'gaze' produces a dichotomous visibility for those subjects, in that their presence acts as a marker for and reflection of their difference; in fact, they can only be present as different. They become identifiable by and identical with their difference. They are subjects who are 'always already given to be seen', subjects characterised by their 'looked-at-ness', subjects semantically marked by their names, identified by their visibility, and fixed by their difference.

To conclude, in response to the assumption that difference is identical with presence, I have suggested, following Derrida, that this presence is mediated by the absence of the 'master signifier'; the primordial, ordering structure. I have argued, therefore, both for an interrogation of difference concepts themselves, and for an interrogation of how and when difference concepts are mobilised.

References

Adams, R., Dominelli, L. and Payne, M. (eds) (1998) *Social Work: Themes, Issues and Critical Debates*, London: Macmillan.

Ahmed, B. (1990) *Black Perspectives in Social Work*, London: Venture Press.

Bonnett, A. (1993) 'The formation of public professional radical consciousness: the example of anti-racism', *Sociology*, vol. 27, no. 2.

Bonnett, A. (2000) *White Identities: Historical and International Perspectives*, Harlow: Prentice Hall.

Braye, S. and Preston-Shoot, M. (1996) *Empowering Practice in Social Care*, Buckingham: Open University Press.

CCETSW (1995) *Paper 30, Rules and Requirements for the Diploma in Social Work*, rev. edn, London: Central Council for Education and Training in Social Work.

Connell, R. (1987) *Gender and Power*, Cambridge: Polity Press.

Cocks, J. (1989) *The Oppositional Imagination: Feminism, Critique and Political Theory*, London: Routledge.

Dalrymple, J. and Burke, B. (1995) *Anti-oppressive Practice: Social Care and the Law*, Buckingham: Open University Press.

Davies, C. and Schleiffer, R. (1991) *Criticism and Culture: the Role of Critique in Modern Literary Theory*, London: Longman.

Dominelli, L. (1999) *Sociology for Social Work*, London: Macmillan.

Dreyfuss, H. and Rabinov, P. (1982) *Michel Foucault: Beyond Structuralism and Hermeneutics*, New York: Harvester Wheatsheaf.

Ely, P. and Denney, D. (1987) *Social Work in a Multi-Racial Society*, Aldershot: Gower.

Foucault, M. (1982) 'The subject and power', Afterword in Dreyfus, H. and Rabinow, P., *Michel Foucault: Beyond Structuralism and Hermeneutics*, Brighton: Harvester.

Fox, N. J. (1998) 'Foucault, Foucauldians and sociology', *British Journal of Sociology*, vol. 49, no. 3.

Fuss, D. (1989) *Essentially Speaking: Feminism, Nature and Difference*, London: Routledge.

Game, A. (1991) *Undoing the Social: Towards a Deconstructive Sociology*, Milton Keynes: Open University.

Gilroy, P. (1987) *There Ain't no Black in the Union Jack*, London: Hutchinson.

Gilroy, P. (1990) 'The end of anti-racism?' *New Community*, vol. 17, no. 1.

Gordon, P. (1991) 'A dirty war: the new right and local authority anti-racism', in Ball, W. and Solomos, J. (eds) *Race and Local Politics*, London: Macmillan.

Grosz, E. (1990) *Jacques Lacan: A Feminist Introduction*, London: Routledge.

Gurnah, A. (1985) 'The politics of racism awareness training', *Critical Social Policy*, vol. 4, no. 2.

Humphries, B. (1997) 'Reading social work: competing discourses in the rules and requirements for the diploma in social work', *British Journal of Social Work*, vol. 27: 641–58.

Jones, C. (1993) 'Distortion and demonisation: the new right and anti-racist social work education', *Social Work Education*, vol. 12. no. 12: 9–16.

Kerfoot, D. and Knights, D. (1994) 'Into the realm of the fearful: power, identity and the gender problematic', in Radtke, L. and Stam, H. J. (eds) *Power! Gender: Social Relations in Theory and Practice*, London: Sage.

Kirton, D. (1995) *Race, Identity and the Politics of Adoption*, University of East London Centre for Adoption and Identity Studies, London: University of East London.

Liff, S. and Wajcman, J. (1996) '"Sameness" and "difference" revisited: which way forward for equal opportunities initiatives?', *Journal of Management Studies*, vol. 33, no.1.

Macey, M. and Moxon, E. (1996) 'An examination of anti-racist and anti-oppressive theory and practice in social work education', *British Journal of Social Work*, vol. 26: 297–314.

Miles, R. (1989) *Racism*, London: Tavistock.

Phillipson, J. (1992) *Practising Equality: Women, Men and Social Work*, London: Central Council for Education and Training in Social Work (CCETSW).

Pinker, R. (1993) 'A lethal kind of looniness', *Times Educational Supplement*, 10 September, London: Times Newspapers.

Preston-Shoot, M. (1995) 'Assessing anti-oppressive practice', *Social Work Education*, vol. 14. no. 2.

Rattansi, A. (1994) '"Western" racisms, ethnicities identities in a "post-modern" frame', in Rattansi, A. and Westwood, S. *Racism, Modernity and Identity on the Western Front*, Cambridge: Polity Press.

Schilling, C. (1993) *The Body and Social Theory*, London: Sage.

Sheshgadri-Crooks, K. (2000) *Desiring Whiteness: A Lacanian Analysis of Race*, London: Routledge.

Singh, G. (1994) 'Political correctness or political change?', *Social Work Education*, vol. 13, no. 5.

Singh, G. (1996) 'Promoting anti-racist and black perspectives in social work education and practice teaching', *Social Work Education*, vol. 15, no. 2.

Sivanandan, A. (1985) 'RAT and the degradation of the black struggle', *Race & Class*, vol. 26, no. 30.

Soja, E. and Hooper, B. (1993) 'The spaces that difference makes: some notes on the geographical margins of the new cultural politics', in Keith, M. and Pile, S. (eds) *Place and the Politics of Identity*, London: Routledge.

Stubbs, P. (1985) 'The employment of black social workers: from "ethnic sensitivity" to anti-racism, *Critical Social Policy*, vol. 4, no. 3.

Thompson, N. (1997) *Anti-Discriminatory Practice*, London: Macmillan.

Trew, W. (1992) *Anti-Racist Strategies and Student Placements: A College Perspective*, London: South Bank University.

Trew, W. (2001) *Anti-Racism in Social Work: In a Cul de Sac or at a Cross Roads?* Unpublished Paper, London: ADP 2000.

Weedon, C. (1987) *Feminist Practice and Post Structuralist Theory*, London: Blackwell.

Author index

Subject index